Larz Trent

AutoRegression
The Journey to the Center of the Self

Original Title: Auto-Regressão: A Jornada para o Centro do Eu
Copyright © 2024, published by Luiz Antonio dos Santos ME. This book is a work of non-fiction that explores practices and concepts in the field of self-knowledge and holistic balance. Through an integrated approach, the author offers practical tools to access the inner essence, promote well-being and cultivate personal transformation.

1st Edition
Production Team
- **Author:** Larz Trent
- **Editor:** Luiz Santos
- **Revision:** Rafael Alencar
- **Cover:** Studios Booklas / Amadeu Rossi
- **Layout:** Clara Mendes
- **Translation:** Hernandez Teles

Publication and Identification
AutoRegression: The Journey to the Center of the Self / By Larz Trent
Editora Booklas, 2024
Categories: Psychology / Personal Development / Self-knowledge
DDC: 158.1 - **CDU:** 159.9

All rights reserved to: Luiz Antonio dos Santos ME / Booklas
No part of this book may be reproduced, stored in a retrieval system, or transmitted by any means — electronic, mechanical, photocopy, [1] recording, or otherwise — without [2] the prior and express permission of the copyright holder.

Summary

Prologue 5
Chapter 1 Journey of Auto-Regression 8
Chapter 2 Unveiling the Holistic System 11
Chapter 3 Vital Energy 14
Chapter 4 Exploring the Dimensions of the Mind 17
Chapter 5 The Mirror of Consciousness 20
Chapter 6 Anchoring in the Present 23
Chapter 7 Awakening Consciousness 26
Chapter 8 Planting the Seeds of Reality 29
Chapter 9 Reprogramming the Subconscious Mind 32
Chapter 10 Identifying Negative Patterns 35
Chapter 11 Emotional Management 38
Chapter 12 Relaxation Techniques 41
Chapter 13 Self-Hypnosis 44
Chapter 14 Awakening Vital Energy 47
Chapter 15 Freeing Yourself from the Past 50
Chapter 16 Cultivating Abundance 53
Chapter 17 Ho'oponopono 56
Chapter 18 Balancing Vital Energy 59
Chapter 19 The Power of Stones in Holistic Healing 62
Chapter 20 Values and Life Purposes 65
Chapter 21 Unleashing Your Unique Potential 68
Chapter 22 Breaking Free from the Chains of Thought 71
Chapter 23 Self-Esteem and Self-Confidence 74

Chapter 24 Assertive Communication 77
Chapter 25 Authentic and Nourishing Connections 80
Chapter 26 Goals and Objectives... 83
Chapter 27 Organizing Your Actions and Resources 87
Chapter 28 Procrastination.. 90
Chapter 29 The Art of Persistence 94
Chapter 30 Resilience 97
Chapter 31 Emotional Intelligence 101
Chapter 32 Unraveling the Mind-Body Connection 105
Chapter 33 Deciphering the Body's Signals.............................. 109
Chapter 34 Self-Regression for Pain Relief............................... 113
Chapter 35 Self-Regression Techniques for Chronic Diseases 117
Chapter 36 Self-Regression and the Immune System............... 121
Chapter 37 Conscious and Intuitive Eating................................ 125
Chapter 38 Conscious Movement 129
Chapter 39 Techniques for Better Sleep 132
Chapter 40 Detoxification of Body and Mind 136
Chapter 41 Hormonal Balance and Self-Regression................. 140
Chapter 42 Self-Regression for Mental Health......................... 144
Chapter 43 Prevention and Health Promotion 148
Chapter 44 Spirituality and Self-Knowledge 152
Chapter 45 Revitalizing Body and Soul...................................... 156
Chapter 46 Developing Intuition... 160
Chapter 47 Synchronicity and the Law of Attraction 164
Chapter 48 Living in Harmony with the Universe..................... 168
Chapter 49 Prosperity and Abundance...................................... 172
Chapter 50 Awakening the Creative Potential.......................... 176

Chapter 51 Expanding the Circle of Love 180
Chapter 52 Awakening Cosmic Consciousness......................... 184
Chapter 53 Living Fully... 188
Chapter 54 A Conscious Lifestyle 192
Chapter 55 Integrating Self-Regression into Life 196
Epilogue 200

Prologue

There is a silent force in this book, something that moves like a subtle but constant current of air, capable of touching every fiber of your consciousness. This is not just another manual, nor a set of practices that promise easy answers. It is, above all, an encounter with the essence that you have often left hidden in layers of conventions and distractions.

As you read it, you will realize that we are not talking about theories. The pages ahead are like trails opened by someone who has already explored this vast territory of self-knowledge and left marks to guide you. Not with shortcuts, but with clues so that each step is conscious, each advance, deeply personal.

And, of all the recommendations I could make, this is perhaps the most important: read this book as someone who allows themselves to be guided by someone who truly cares about the impact each word will have on your life. Here, you will find tools that are not only useful, but essential to open doors that you may not even know existed within you.

The text is not imposing, nor condescending. It speaks to you as a mentor who sees potential where you only see limits, and who challenges you to take a step beyond what you think is possible. There is something extraordinary about discovering that, in the practice of auto-regression, what you are really looking for is not something new, but what has always been there - waiting to be recognized, transformed and integrated.

There is an almost surgical precision in the approaches presented here. With each page, you will be invited to identify what has been blocking your growth, to question the beliefs you hold, often without even realizing it, and to find a harmonious flow between body, mind and spirit. This is not a superficial experience; it is a deeply regenerative journey.

I recommend, above all, that you read with curiosity, with an open mind and with a genuine willingness to allow yourself to be touched. With each suggested exercise, don't just think about how to apply it, but feel the transformation it can bring. This is not advice from a theorist, but from someone who sees the real impact this work can have on the life of anyone who dedicates themselves to it.

Finally, allow me a provocation. If there is a part of you that hesitates to surrender to what this book proposes, it is precisely because there is something valuable waiting to be awakened. There is no urgency, but there is a silent promise that, as you progress through these pages, you will discover something that will resonate far beyond reading.

Accept this invitation, not because you need to, but because you deserve to.

Luiz Santos

Editor

Chapter 1
Journey of Auto-Regression

Imagine a garden. In it, you find vibrant flowers, succulent fruits and aromatic herbs. But there are also weeds, dry branches and stones that prevent full bloom. This garden is you, a complete being with potentialities and limitations. Auto-regression is the art of cultivating this inner garden, removing obstacles and nurturing the seeds of your well-being.

Auto-regression is a journey of self-knowledge and transformation. It is the ability to look at yourself with honesty and compassion, to recognize your emotions, thoughts and behaviors, and to take responsibility for your own life. It is an active process of healing and growth, which empowers you to walk a path of self-discovery and fulfillment.

On this path, you will learn to identify and reframe limiting patterns, negative beliefs and trapped emotions. You will discover the power of internal dialogue and the importance of cultivating positive and constructive thoughts. You will learn to master your emotions, free yourself from the past and build healthier relationships.

Auto-regression invites you to dive into yourself, to explore the depths of your being and to connect with your essence. It is a process of self-healing that allows you to access inner resources and awaken dormant potentials.

Through auto-regression, you can:

Increase your self-awareness: Understand your thoughts, feelings and behaviors, and how they impact your life.

Manage your emotions: Learn to deal with stress, anxiety, anger and other challenging emotions.

- Overcome limiting beliefs: Identify and transform beliefs that prevent you from achieving your goals.
- Improve your relationships: Build healthier and more authentic relationships.
- Achieve your goals: Set goals and create strategies to achieve what you want.
- Raise your self-esteem: Develop self-love and confidence in yourself.
- Live with more purpose: Find meaning and direction in your life.
- Awaken your intuition: Connect with your inner wisdom.
- Cultivate inner peace: Find serenity and balance amidst life's challenges.

Auto-regression is a powerful tool to transform your life. It is an invitation to take control of your destiny and create the reality you desire. It is a journey of healing, growth and self-discovery, which will lead you to a fuller, more authentic and happier life.

Exercise:

Take a moment to reflect on the following questions:
- What motivates you to seek auto-regression?
- What areas of your life would you like to transform?
- What are your biggest challenges and how can auto-regression help you overcome them?

Write down your answers in a journal and revisit them throughout your journey of self-knowledge.

Auto-regression is an ongoing process of learning and growth. Be patient with yourself, celebrate each step taken and trust in your ability to transform. You are the protagonist of your story and have the power to create the life you have always dreamed of.

Chapter 2
Unveiling the Holistic System

Imagine the human being as a complex and interconnected system, composed of body, mind and spirit. Each part influences and is influenced by the others, forming a dynamic and inseparable web. The holistic system recognizes this interdependence and seeks harmony between all dimensions of being.

The Physical Body: It is the dwelling place of our soul, the vehicle that allows us to experience the world. Taking care of the body with healthy eating, physical exercise and relaxation practices is fundamental for general well-being. However, the physical body is only part of the story.

The Mind: It is the seat of our thoughts, emotions and beliefs. It is the mind that interprets the world, creates our reality and shapes our experiences. A serene and balanced mind is essential for health and happiness.

The Spirit: It is our essence, the divine spark that connects us with something greater than ourselves. It is the source of our intuition, creativity and life purpose. Nurturing the spirit with practices such as meditation, contact with nature and connection with spirituality allows us to access inner wisdom and live with more meaning.

In the holistic system, disease is not seen only as a physical problem, but as an imbalance in the whole system. Repressed emotions, negative thoughts and lack of spiritual connection can manifest as physical symptoms. Likewise, health is not just the absence of disease, but the integral well-being of body, mind and spirit.

Auto-regression, in this context, acts as a catalyst for harmony. Through techniques and practices, it helps us identify and transform patterns of thought and behavior that generate imbalances, promoting healing and well-being at all levels.

Understanding the interaction between body, mind and spirit:
- **Emotions and physical health:** Emotions such as stress, anxiety and anger can affect the immune system, blood pressure and the functioning of organs.
- **Thoughts and well-being:** Negative thoughts and limiting beliefs can generate anxiety, depression and other mental health problems.
- **Spirituality and healing:** Connection with spirituality can promote inner peace, hope and optimism, helping in the recovery from illness and in coping with challenges.

Exercise:
Observe how your thoughts, emotions and physical sensations manifest themselves in different situations of your daily life.
- When you feel stressed, what are your body's reactions?

- How do your thoughts influence your emotions?
- How does your spirituality contribute to your well-being?

Write down your observations and reflect on how you can cultivate harmony between body, mind and spirit.

You are an integral being, a complex and interconnected system. By taking care of all dimensions of your being, you pave the way for a healthier, more balanced and fulfilling life. Auto-regression invites you to take responsibility for your health and well-being, and to walk a path of self-knowledge and transformation.

Chapter 3
Vital Energy

In the previous chapters, we explored self-regression as a path to self-knowledge and the holistic system as the fertile ground where this journey unfolds. Now, let's dive into one of the fundamental pillars of this journey: vital energy.

Imagine vital energy as a river flowing through your being, nourishing every cell, every organ, every thought and emotion. This energy, known in various cultures as Chi, Prana or Ki, is the vital force that animates the body, mind and spirit.

Just as a river can be blocked by rocks and debris, vital energy can also encounter obstacles in its path. Negative emotions, past traumas, limiting beliefs and harmful habits can create energy blocks, preventing the free flow of vital energy and affecting health and well-being.

Self-regression, in this context, acts as a tool to remove these blocks and restore the harmonious flow of vital energy. Through techniques such as meditation, conscious breathing, visualization and energy practices, you can learn to release stagnant energy, revitalize the body and mind, and awaken inner strength.

Understanding energy centers:

In the holistic system, vital energy flows through subtle channels in the body known as meridians. Along these meridians, we find centers of concentrated energy, called chakras. Each chakra is associated with different aspects of the human being, such as emotions, physical health and spiritual development.

- **Root Chakra:** Located at the base of the spine, it is linked to security, stability and connection to the earth.
- **Sacral Chakra:** Located below the navel, it is related to creativity, sexuality and pleasure.
- **Solar Plexus Chakra:** Located in the stomach area, it is associated with personal power, self-esteem and self-confidence.
- **Heart Chakra:** Located in the center of the chest, it is linked to love, compassion and connection with others.
- **Throat Chakra:** Located in the throat, it is related to communication, expression and creativity.
- **Third Eye Chakra:** Located on the forehead, between the eyebrows, it is associated with intuition, wisdom and inner vision.
- **Crown Chakra:** Located at the top of the head, it is linked to spirituality, connection with the divine and transcendence.

When the chakras are balanced and harmonized, vital energy flows freely, promoting health, vitality and well-being. Blockages in one or more chakras can generate emotional, physical and spiritual imbalances.

Exercise:

Pay attention to how you feel about each of the chakras.
- Do you feel safe and connected to the earth?
- Do you express your creativity and sexuality freely?
- Do you feel confident and empowered?
- Do you cultivate love and compassion in your relationships?
- Do you communicate with clarity and authenticity?
- Do you trust your intuition and follow your inner vision?
- Do you feel connected to something greater than yourself?

Reflect on how you can balance and harmonize your chakras through self-regression.

Vital energy is the force that animates life. By learning to cultivate and harmonize this energy, you awaken your potential for healing and transformation. Self-regression invites you to connect with this inner strength and to walk a path of self-discovery and fulfillment.

Chapter 4
Exploring the Dimensions of the Mind

So far, we have explored self-regression, the holistic system and the vital energy that permeates our being. In this chapter, we will enter the fascinating world of states of consciousness, the different ways in which our mind perceives and interacts with reality.

Imagine consciousness as a spectrum of light, with infinite nuances and gradations. At each moment, our mind is in a specific state of consciousness, which influences our perception, emotions, thoughts and behaviors.

The most common state of consciousness is the waking state, the one in which we are awake and interacting with the external world. In this state, our senses are alert, our mind is focused on the present and we are aware of ourselves and the environment around us.

However, there are other states of consciousness that we can access, each with its own characteristics and potentials. Sleep, for example, is an altered state of consciousness in which the body rests and the mind disconnects from the outside world. During sleep, we go through different phases, including REM sleep, where dreams occur.

In addition to sleep, there are other altered states of consciousness, such as trance, hypnosis and meditation. In these states, the mind becomes still, attention turns inward and we can access deeper levels of consciousness.

Self-regression allows us to explore and expand our states of consciousness. Through techniques such as meditation, relaxation and visualization, we can learn to control our brain waves, deepen our connection with our inner self and access higher states of consciousness.

Expanding consciousness:
- **Beta State:** It is the waking state, characterized by rapid brain waves and intense mental activity. In this state, we are alert, focused and ready to act.
- **Alpha State:** It is a state of light relaxation, where brain waves become slower. In this state, the mind is calm, creative and receptive to new ideas.
- **Theta State:** It is a state of deep relaxation, where brain waves are even slower. In this state, we can access the subconscious, release blocked emotions and memories, and have deep insights.
- **Delta State:** It is the state of deep sleep, where brain waves are very slow. In this state, the body regenerates and the mind rests completely.
- **Gamma State:** It is a state of high brain frequency, associated with intuition, insights and mystical experiences. In this state, the mind is highly focused and connected to an expanded consciousness.

Exercise:

Experiment with different relaxation and meditation techniques to access deeper states of consciousness. Observe how your mind and body react to each technique. What sensations do you experience? What thoughts and emotions arise?

Self-regression invites you to explore the different dimensions of your mind and expand your consciousness. By accessing higher states of consciousness, you can awaken your potential for healing, creativity and self-knowledge. The journey of self-regression is a fascinating adventure into the unknown, an exploration of the infinite possibilities of your mind.

Chapter 5
The Mirror of Consciousness

Imagine a mirror that reflects not only your outer image, but also your deepest thoughts, emotions and behaviors. Self-observation is that mirror, a powerful tool that allows you to observe yourself with clarity and honesty, without judgments or criticism.

Through self-observation, you become aware of your thought patterns, your emotional reactions and your behavioral habits. You begin to realize how your thoughts influence your emotions, how your emotions affect your actions and how your actions shape your reality.

Self-observation is like a light that illuminates the dark corners of your mind, revealing limiting beliefs, fears and insecurities that may be preventing you from living fully. By bringing these patterns to consciousness, you can begin to transform them and create a more authentic and happy life.

Developing self-observation:
- **Pay attention to your thoughts:** Observe the constant flow of thoughts that pass through your mind. What are the recurring themes? What are the beliefs that support these thoughts?

- **Identify your emotions:** Pay attention to your emotional reactions in different situations. What makes you feel happy, sad, anxious or irritated? How do you express your emotions?
- **Observe your behaviors:** Analyze your habits and actions. How do you react to challenges? How do you relate to other people? What are your behavior patterns?
- **Write down your observations:** Keep a journal to record your thoughts, emotions and behaviors. This practice will help you identify patterns and track your progress on the journey of self-knowledge.
- **Practice meditation:** Meditation is a powerful tool for developing self-observation. By stilling the mind and observing your thoughts without judgment, you cultivate mental clarity and self-awareness.

The benefits of self-observation:
- **Self-knowledge:** Understand your thoughts, emotions and behaviors.
- **Emotional management:** Learn to deal with your emotions more effectively.
- **Personal transformation:** Identify and change thought and behavior patterns that no longer serve you.
- **Improved relationships:** Communicate more clearly and authentically.
- **Stress reduction:** Learn to observe your thoughts and emotions without identifying with them.

- **Increased self-compassion:** Develop a kind and understanding attitude towards yourself.

Exercise:

Spend a few minutes each day observing your thoughts and emotions without judgment. Simply observe what is happening in your mind and body. Write down your observations in a journal.

Self-observation is a skill that develops with practice. Be patient with yourself and celebrate each step taken on the journey of self-knowledge. By observing yourself with clarity and honesty, you pave the way for personal transformation and a fuller and more authentic life.

Chapter 6
Anchoring in the Present

Imagine your breath as a bridge connecting your body and mind. With each inhale, you absorb vital energy and oxygen, nourishing every cell of your being. With each exhale, you release toxins and tensions, purifying your body and calming your mind.

Breathing is an automatic and essential process for life, but it often goes unnoticed. However, by paying attention to your breath, you anchor yourself in the present moment, calm the whirlwind of thoughts, and connect with your body and emotions.

Conscious breathing is a simple but powerful practice that can be used anytime, anywhere. It helps you deal with stress, anxiety, and other challenging emotions, in addition to promoting relaxation, concentration, and overall well-being.

Exploring conscious breathing:
- **Observe your breath:** Sit in a comfortable position and close your eyes. Pay attention to the natural movement of your breath, without trying to control it. Notice the air entering and leaving your lungs, the movement of your abdomen and chest.

- **Breathe deeply:** Inhale slowly and deeply through your nose, expanding your abdomen and filling your lungs with air. Exhale slowly through your mouth, emptying your lungs and contracting your abdomen.
- **Count your breaths:** Inhale counting to four, hold the air counting to four, exhale counting to four, and hold the air counting to four. Repeat this cycle for a few minutes.
- **Practice alternate breathing:** Sit in a comfortable position and close your eyes. With your right thumb, close your right nostril and inhale through your left nostril. Close your left nostril with your right ring finger and exhale through your right nostril. Inhale through your right nostril, close it [1] with your right thumb, and exhale through your left nostril. Continue alternating nostrils for a few minutes.

The benefits of conscious breathing:
- **Stress and anxiety reduction:** Deep, slow breathing calms the nervous system and reduces the production of stress hormones.
- **Improved concentration:** Conscious breathing helps you focus on the present moment and calm the mind.
- **Increased self-awareness:** By paying attention to your breath, you become more aware of your body and your emotions.

- **Improved physical health:** Deep breathing increases blood oxygenation and promotes muscle relaxation.
- **Emotional balance:** Conscious breathing helps you deal with challenging emotions such as anger, fear, and sadness.

Exercise:

Practice conscious breathing for a few minutes every day. You can do this when you wake up, before bed, or anytime you need to calm down and connect with the present moment.

Breathing is an anchor that connects you to the here and now. By cultivating conscious breathing, you become more present, more aware, and more connected to your inner being. Breathing is a gift you can give yourself at any moment, a path to inner peace and well-being.

Chapter 7
Awakening Consciousness

Imagine a lake agitated by the waves of thought, emotions, and worries. Meditation is like the calm that sets in after the storm, allowing the water to calm down and reflect the beauty of the sky.

Meditation is a practice that involves concentrating attention on a single point, such as the breath, a mantra, or an image. By focusing the mind, thoughts dissipate, mental agitation calms down, and consciousness expands.

Mindfulness, in turn, is the practice of paying attention to the present moment without judgment. It is observing your thoughts, emotions, and physical sensations with acceptance and curiosity, without getting carried away by them.

Unraveling meditation and mindfulness:
- **Find a quiet place:** Choose a calm environment free from distractions to practice meditation.
- **Sit comfortably:** Find a comfortable position with your spine straight and your shoulders relaxed.
- **Close your eyes:** Close your eyes to reduce visual distractions and turn your attention inward.

- **Focus on your breath:** Pay attention to the natural movement of your breath, observing the air entering and leaving your lungs.
- **Observe your thoughts:** When thoughts arise, observe them without judgment, like clouds passing across the sky. Don't cling to them, just let them go and return your attention to your breath.
- **Practice guided meditation:** Use guided meditations to help you with the process of concentration and relaxation.
- **Incorporate mindfulness into your daily life:** Pay attention to your senses during everyday activities, such as eating, walking, or taking a bath. Observe the flavors, smells, textures, and sensations with full attention.

The benefits of meditation and mindfulness:
- **Stress and anxiety reduction:** Calms the mind and body, reducing the production of stress hormones.
- **Improved concentration and focus:** Strengthens attention and the ability to concentrate.
- **Increased self-awareness:** Promotes connection with your inner self and understanding of your thoughts and emotions.
- **Cultivation of compassion and empathy:** Develops the ability to connect with others and understand their perspectives.
- **Improved mental and physical health:** Strengthens the immune system, reduces blood pressure, and improves sleep quality.

- **Increased creativity and intuition:** Opens the mind to new ideas and insights.
- **Cultivation of inner peace:** Promotes serenity, acceptance, and connection with the present moment.

Exercise:

Start with small meditation practices, 5 to 10 minutes a day. Use apps or videos with guided meditations to help you through the process. Incorporate mindfulness into your daily activities, paying attention to your senses and the present moment.

Meditation and mindfulness are like muscles that are strengthened with practice. Be patient with yourself, celebrate each step taken, and trust the process. By quieting the mind and cultivating presence, you pave the way for a fuller, more conscious, and happier life.

Chapter 8
Planting the Seeds of Reality

In the previous chapters, we have traveled a path that has taken us from self-regression to the holistic system, from vital energy to states of consciousness, from self-observation to conscious breathing and meditation. Now, let's explore the power of creative visualization, a technique that allows us to use our imagination to create the reality we desire.

Imagine an artist who, with his paints and brushes, brings a blank canvas to life. Creative visualization is like that art, where you use the power of your mind to create vivid and detailed images of what you want to manifest in your life.

Creative visualization is much more than just "positive thinking". It is an active and conscious process of using imagination, emotions, and energy to create a clear and detailed mental representation of your goal, as if it were already real.

By visualizing with clarity and emotion, you send a powerful message to your subconscious, which in turn begins to work to attract the circumstances, people, and resources needed to fulfill your desire.

Mastering the art of creative visualization:
- **Define your goal:** What do you really want to manifest in your life? Be specific and clear when defining your goal.
- **Create a mental image:** Close your eyes and imagine your goal as if it were already real. Visualize with as much detail as possible: colors, shapes, sounds, smells, sensations.
- **Engage your emotions:** Feel the joy, gratitude, and satisfaction of having already achieved your goal. The more emotion you put into visualization, the more powerful it will be.
- **Affirm your desire:** Repeat positive affirmations that reinforce the achievement of your goal. Use phrases in the present tense, such as "I am grateful for having achieved..." or "I am living...".
- **Practice regularly:** Set aside time each day to practice creative visualization. The more you practice, the easier it will be to create vivid and detailed images.
- **Trust the process:** Believe that your goal is manifesting in your life. Maintain a positive and confident attitude.

The benefits of creative visualization:
- **Goal achievement:** Helps to manifest your dreams and desires.
- **Increased self-esteem:** Strengthens belief in yourself and your ability to create the reality you want.
- **Improved health:** Can be used to promote healing and physical well-being.

- **Overcoming challenges:** Helps to deal with difficult situations and find creative solutions.
- **Increased creativity:** Stimulates imagination and the ability to create new ideas.
- **Improved performance:** Can be used to improve performance in various areas, such as sports, studies, and work.

Exercise:

Choose a goal you want to achieve and practice creative visualization for a few minutes every day. Imagine your goal as if it were already real, engaging your emotions and affirming your desire.

Creative visualization is a powerful tool for creating the reality you desire. By using your imagination, your emotions, and your energy, you plant the seeds of your reality and reap the fruits of your dreams.

Chapter 9
Reprogramming the Subconscious Mind

Imagine your mind as a garden. If you plant flower seeds, you will have a flower garden. If you plant weeds, you will have an infested garden. Positive affirmations are like seeds that you plant in your mind. By repeating positive and inspiring phrases, you cultivate thoughts and beliefs that propel you towards your goals.

The subconscious is like fertile soil that absorbs everything you plant in it. If you feed your mind with negative thoughts, fears, and insecurities, you will be cultivating a barren ground for your dreams. But if you nurture your mind with positive affirmations, you will be creating an environment conducive to growth and fulfillment.

Positive affirmations are short, powerful phrases that express what you want to manifest in your life. By repeating them with conviction and emotion, you send a clear message to your subconscious, which in turn begins to work to align your reality with your desires.

Mastering the Power of Affirmations:
- **Choose affirmations that resonate with you:** Select phrases that express your desires and goals clearly and positively.

- **Use the present tense:** Formulate your affirmations as if what you desire is already real. For example, instead of saying "I want to be happy", say "I am happy".
- **Repeat your affirmations frequently:** Repeat your affirmations several times a day, aloud or mentally.
- **Put emotion into your affirmations:** Feel the emotion of already having achieved what you desire when repeating your affirmations.
- **Write your affirmations:** Write your affirmations in a notebook or on cards and place them in visible places, such as on the bathroom mirror or refrigerator.
- **Create a positive environment:** Surround yourself with people, books, movies, and music that inspire and motivate you.

The Benefits of Positive Affirmations:
- **Mental reprogramming:** Replaces negative thoughts with positive ones.
- **Increased self-esteem:** Strengthens belief in yourself and your abilities.
- **Goal achievement:** Helps you achieve your dreams and desires.
- **Improved health:** Promotes physical and mental well-being.
- **Overcoming challenges:** Strengthens resilience and the ability to deal with difficulties.
- **Increased motivation:** Inspires and drives action.

Exercise:

Create a list of positive affirmations that express your desires and goals. Repeat them frequently, with conviction and emotion. Observe how your thoughts and feelings change over time.

Positive affirmations are powerful tools for reprogramming your mind and creating the reality you desire. By planting seeds of positivity in your mental garden, you reap the fruits of a happier, more abundant, and fulfilling life.

Chapter 10
Identifying Negative Patterns

In previous chapters, we explored powerful tools of self-regression, such as creative visualization and positive affirmations. Now, let's delve deeper into the internal dialogue, that constant conversation we have with ourselves, and learn to identify and transform negative patterns that may be limiting our potential.

Imagine your mind as a stage where your thoughts are the main actors. Internal dialogue is the play that is always showing, with lines, scenery, and characters that repeat day after day. If the play is negative, with critical dialogues, dark scenarios, and defeatist characters, the result will be a life marked by insecurities, fears, and frustrations.

But if you rewrite the script, transform negative lines into positive ones, dark scenarios into inspiring scenarios, and defeatist characters into confident characters, your life will be transformed into a journey of self-knowledge, empowerment, and fulfillment.

Negative self-talk is like a virus that takes hold in our minds, undermining our self-esteem, sabotaging our dreams, and preventing us from living fully. It manifests in the form of criticism, judgments, doubts, and fears, and can stem from past experiences, limiting beliefs, and dysfunctional thought patterns.

Identifying and Transforming Negative Self-Talk:
- **Pay attention to your inner voice:** Notice the thoughts that arise in your mind throughout the day. What are the recurring themes? What are the words and phrases you use to refer to yourself?
- **Identify negative patterns:** What are the limiting beliefs that fuel your negative self-talk? Do you criticize yourself frequently? Do you doubt your abilities? Do you compare yourself to others?
- **Question your thoughts:** When a negative thought arises, question its validity. Is it really true? Is there evidence to support it? What are the other possible perspectives?
- **Rewrite the script:** Replace negative thoughts with positive and empowering affirmations. Instead of saying "I am not capable", say "I am capable of achieving my dreams".
- **Cultivate self-compassion:** Treat yourself with kindness and understanding, as you would a dear friend. Forgive yourself for your mistakes and acknowledge your qualities and achievements.
- **Practice gratitude:** Focus on the good things in your life and be thankful for them. Gratitude is a powerful antidote to negativity.

The Benefits of Transforming Self-Talk:
- **Increased self-esteem:** Strengthens confidence in yourself and your abilities.

- **Improved mental health:** Reduces anxiety, depression, and stress.
- **Goal achievement:** Increases motivation and persistence in pursuit of your dreams.
- **Improved relationships:** Promotes assertive communication and empathy.
- **Increased happiness:** Cultivates optimism, gratitude, and inner peace.

Exercise:

Write down your negative thoughts in a journal and then rewrite them in a positive and empowering way. Practice self-observation and each time a negative thought arises, question it and replace it with a positive affirmation.

You have the power to transform your inner dialogue and create a more positive and empowering reality. By rewriting the script of your mind, you become the author of your own story and the protagonist of your life.

Chapter 11
Emotional Management

Imagine emotions as wild horses, full of energy and vitality. If you don't know how to tame them, they can take you down unexpected and even dangerous paths. But if you learn to lead them with wisdom and firmness, they will take you where you want to go, with strength and determination.

Emotional management is not about repressing or denying emotions, but about welcoming them, understanding them, and directing them constructively. It is learning to recognize the signals that emotions send us, to identify the triggers that trigger them, and to develop strategies to deal with them in a healthy and balanced way.

Emotions such as joy, sadness, anger, fear, and love are part of the human experience and play a fundamental role in our lives. They provide us with important information about ourselves and the world around us, motivate us to act, and connect us with others.

However, when emotions are intense, uncontrolled, or repressed, they can generate suffering, conflict, and imbalance. Emotional management allows us to navigate the waves of emotions with more serenity, balance, and wisdom.

Developing Emotional Intelligence:
- **Emotional self-awareness:** Pay attention to your emotions, identify them, and name them. Notice how they manifest in your body and thoughts.
- **Understanding emotions:** Seek to understand the origin of your emotions, the triggers that trigger them, and the messages they bring.
- **Acceptance of emotions:** Welcome your emotions without judgment, recognizing that they are part of your human experience.
- **Emotional regulation:** Develop strategies to deal with intense emotions, such as mindful breathing, meditation, physical exercise, and assertive communication.
- **Emotional expression:** Express your emotions authentically and respectfully, using non-violent communication and active listening.
- **Empathy:** Cultivate the ability to put yourself in another's shoes and understand their emotions.

Benefits of Emotional Management:
- **Mental and emotional well-being:** Reduces anxiety, stress, and depression.
- **Improved relationships:** Promotes effective communication, empathy, and conflict resolution.
- **Increased self-esteem:** Strengthens self-confidence and self-acceptance.
- **Goal achievement:** Increases motivation, persistence, and the ability to deal with frustrations.

- **Improved physical health:** Reduces the risk of heart disease, improves the immune system, and promotes overall well-being.

Exercise:

Identify an emotion that you have difficulty dealing with. Notice how it manifests in your body and thoughts. Try to understand the origin of this emotion and the triggers that trigger it. Develop strategies to deal with this emotion in a healthy and balanced way.

Emotions are like compasses that guide us through life. By learning to master them, you become the captain of your ship, sailing safely and wisely towards your goals. Emotional management is a journey of self-knowledge, empowerment, and inner freedom.

Chapter 12
Relaxation Techniques

In the previous chapters, we explored the power of emotional management and learned to master the reins of our inner experience. Now, let's dive into a set of relaxation techniques that help us calm the body and mind, promoting well-being and balance amidst life's challenges.

Imagine a rough sea, with choppy waves and strong winds. Relaxation techniques are like a beacon that guides your boat towards calm and tranquil waters, where you can rest and recharge your energies.

Stress, anxiety, and the tensions of everyday life can accumulate in our body and mind, generating symptoms such as muscle aches, insomnia, irritability, and difficulty concentrating. Relaxation techniques are powerful tools to release these tensions, restore balance, and promote physical and mental health.

There are several relaxation techniques, each with its benefits and particularities. Some techniques focus on muscle relaxation, others on breathing, and others on visualization and meditation. The important thing is to find the techniques that best suit your needs and preferences and incorporate them into your daily routine.

Exploring Relaxation Techniques:
- **Progressive muscle relaxation:** This technique consists of tensing and relaxing different muscle groups, promoting body awareness and deep relaxation.
- **Diaphragmatic breathing:** Deep, slow breathing, using the diaphragm, calms the nervous system and reduces anxiety.
- **Meditation:** The practice of meditation calms the mind, reduces stress, and promotes inner peace.
- **Yoga:** The practice of yoga combines physical postures, breathing exercises, and meditation, promoting relaxation, flexibility, and well-being.
- **Massage:** Massage relaxes muscles, relieves tension, and promotes blood circulation.
- **Aromatherapy:** The use of essential oils with relaxing properties, such as lavender and chamomile, can help relieve stress and anxiety.
- **Relaxing music:** Listening to soft, instrumental music can calm the mind and promote relaxation.
- **Hot bath:** A hot bath with relaxing bath salts can relieve muscle tension and promote well-being.

Benefits of Relaxation Techniques:
- **Reduction of stress and anxiety:** Calms the nervous system and reduces the production of stress hormones.
- **Improved sleep quality:** Promotes relaxation and makes it easier to fall asleep.
- **Relief of muscle aches and tension:** Relaxes muscles and relieves pain.

- **Improved concentration and focus:** Calms the mind and increases mental clarity.
- **Increased self-awareness:** Promotes connection with the body and emotions.
- **Improved physical and mental health:** Strengthens the immune system, reduces blood pressure, and promotes general well-being.

Exercise:

Try different relaxation techniques and find the ones that benefit you the most. Incorporate them into your daily routine, taking a few minutes each day to relax and recharge your batteries.

Relaxation techniques are like tools that help you navigate the turbulent waters of life with more serenity and balance. By calming the body and mind, you make room for inner peace, health, and well-being.

Chapter 13
Self-Hypnosis

In the previous chapters, we explored various techniques to calm the mind and body, such as relaxation and meditation. Now, let's enter the fascinating world of self-hypnosis, a powerful tool for accessing the subconscious and reprogramming beliefs, habits, and behaviors.

Imagine the mind as an iceberg, where the visible part represents the conscious mind and the submerged part, much larger, represents the subconscious. Self-hypnosis is like a deep dive into this inner ocean, allowing you to access the depths of your mind and explore your unlimited potential.

Hypnosis is a natural state of altered consciousness, characterized by an intense focus of attention and increased receptivity to suggestions. During self-hypnosis, you induce this state in yourself, guiding your mind to a state of deep relaxation and concentration.

In this state, the subconscious becomes more accessible, allowing you to plant new ideas, beliefs, and behaviors that align with your goals and desires. Self-hypnosis can be used for a variety of purposes, such as overcoming fears and phobias, eliminating unwanted habits, increasing self-esteem, improving performance, and promoting physical and emotional healing.

Mastering the Art of Self-Hypnosis:
- **Find a quiet place:** Choose a calm environment free from distractions to practice self-hypnosis.
- **Adopt a comfortable posture:** Sit or lie down in a relaxing position, with your spine straight and your muscles relaxed.
- **Induce relaxation:** Use relaxation techniques, such as deep breathing and progressive muscle relaxation, to calm the body and mind.
- **Focus your attention:** Focus your attention on a fixed point, such as an image, an object, or your own breathing.
- **Use positive suggestions:** Create short, positive phrases that express what you want to achieve, such as "I am confident", "I am at peace" or "I am able to overcome my challenges".
- **Repeat the suggestions:** Repeat the suggestions mentally or in a low voice, with conviction and emotion.
- **Visualize your goals:** Imagine yourself achieving your goals, experiencing the emotions and sensations as if they were already real.
- **Exit the hypnotic state:** When you are ready to come out of the hypnotic state, count from 1 to 5, gradually opening your eyes and returning to your normal consciousness.

Benefits of Self-Hypnosis:

- **Mental reprogramming:** Allows you to reprogram limiting beliefs and install new patterns of thought and behavior.
- **Overcoming fears and phobias:** Helps to deal with fears and phobias, such as fear of public speaking, fear of heights, or fear of animals.
- **Eliminating unwanted habits:** Helps in eliminating habits such as smoking, biting nails, or overeating.
- **Increased self-esteem:** Strengthens self-confidence and self-acceptance.
- **Improved performance:** Increases concentration, focus, and motivation to achieve your goals.
- **Promoting healing:** Assists in the healing of physical and emotional illnesses, such as chronic pain, anxiety, and depression.

Exercise:

Try a self-hypnosis session guided by a professional or use a self-hypnosis app. Create your own positive suggestions and repeat them with conviction and emotion. Visualize your goals as if they were already real.

Self-hypnosis is a powerful tool for accessing your inner potential and creating the life you desire. By diving into the depths of your mind, you can reprogram your beliefs, overcome your limits, and manifest your dreams.

Chapter 14
Awakening Vital Energy

Imagine the body as a river, where vital energy flows freely, nourishing every cell and organ. Yoga and stretching are like movements that remove obstacles in this river, allowing vital energy to circulate freely, revitalizing the body and mind.

Yoga is an ancient practice that combines physical postures (asanas), breathing exercises (pranayamas), and meditation, promoting the union between body, mind, and spirit. Through asanas, yoga stretches and strengthens muscles, increases flexibility, improves posture, and stimulates the flow of vital energy.

Stretching, in turn, is a practice that aims to increase the flexibility and range of motion of the joints, preventing injuries, relieving muscle aches, and promoting relaxation.

Awakening Vital Energy Through Yoga and Stretching:
- **Find a quiet space:** Choose a calm environment free from distractions to practice yoga or stretching.
- **Wear comfortable clothes:** Wear clothes that allow free movement of the body.

- **Start with basic postures:** If you are new to yoga, start with basic postures and gradually progress.
- **Breathe consciously:** Pay attention to your breathing during practice, inhaling and exhaling deeply.
- **Listen to your body:** Respect your limits and don't force your body beyond what it can handle.
- **Practice regularly:** Regular practice of yoga and stretching brings more benefits than sporadic practice.
- **Combine postures and stretches:** Try combining different yoga postures with specific stretches for each muscle group.
- **Explore different styles of yoga:** There are several styles of yoga, such as Hatha Yoga, Vinyasa Yoga, Ashtanga Yoga, and Iyengar Yoga. Try different styles and find the one that best suits your needs and preferences.

Benefits of Yoga and Stretching:

- **Increased flexibility and strength:** Improves flexibility, muscle strength, and physical endurance.
- **Improved posture:** Corrects posture, aligns the spine, and prevents back pain.
- **Reduced stress and anxiety:** Calms the nervous system and reduces the production of stress hormones.
- **Improved blood circulation:** Stimulates blood and lymphatic circulation, oxygenating tissues and eliminating toxins.

- **Increased vital energy:** Unblocks energy channels and promotes the free flow of vital energy.
- **Improved concentration and focus:** Calms the mind and increases mental clarity.
- **Increased self-awareness:** Promotes connection with the body and physical sensations.
- **Improved physical and mental health:** Strengthens the immune system, prevents diseases, and promotes general well-being.

Exercise:

Start practicing yoga or stretching with a basic sequence of postures. Pay attention to your breathing and your limits. Try different styles of yoga and find the one you like best.

Yoga and stretching are like dances that celebrate life and the vital energy that flows in our body. By integrating these practices into your routine, you cultivate health, balance, and harmony between body, mind, and spirit.

Chapter 15
Freeing Yourself from the Past

In the previous chapters, we learned to care for our physical body as a temple of vital energy. Now, let's turn to emotional healing and explore the art of forgiveness, a powerful balm for the wounds of the past.

Imagine forgiveness as a key that opens the doors of a prison where you keep the hurts, resentments, and pains of the past imprisoned. By forgiving, you free yourself from these chains, opening space for healing, inner peace, and emotional freedom.

Forgiving does not mean forgetting or denying what happened, nor justifying the actions of those who hurt you. Forgiving is, above all, an act of self-love, a conscious choice to free yourself from the weight of the past and move forward with lightness and serenity.

When we cling to anger, resentment, and hurt, we are holding ourselves to the past and preventing emotional wounds from healing. Forgiveness, on the other hand, frees us from this emotional prison, allowing vital energy to flow freely and healing to happen on all levels of our being.

The path of forgiveness:
- **Acknowledge your emotions:** Allow yourself to feel anger, sadness, hurt, and all the emotions that

arise when you remember the situation that hurt you. Don't suppress your emotions, embrace them with compassion and understanding.
- **Identify the need behind the emotion:** Ask yourself, "What do I need to feel at peace with this situation?". Perhaps you need acknowledgment, an apology, justice, or simply time to heal.
- **Cultivate empathy:** Try to put yourself in the shoes of the person who hurt you and understand their motivations and their pain. This does not mean justifying their actions, but rather developing compassion and understanding.
- **Make the decision to forgive:** Forgiveness is a conscious choice, an act of will. Decide to forgive yourself and others, freeing yourself from the weight of the past.
- **Practice forgiveness daily:** Forgiveness is a process that takes time and practice. Repeat affirmations of forgiveness, visualize the situation that hurt you, and imagine yourself forgiving with love and compassion.
- **Free yourself from the past:** Focus on the present and the future, building a life free of hurts and resentments.

The benefits of forgiveness:
- **Emotional liberation:** Frees you from the weight of the past and negative emotions.
- **Emotional healing:** Promotes the healing of emotional wounds and overcoming trauma.

- **Improved relationships:** Restores relationships and promotes reconciliation.
- **Increased inner peace:** Cultivates serenity, harmony, and emotional well-being.
- **Improved physical health:** Reduces stress, anxiety, and related physical symptoms.
- **Increased compassion and empathy:** Develops the ability to forgive and understand yourself and others.

Exercise:

Write a letter to the person who hurt you, expressing your feelings and your decision to forgive. It is not necessary to send the letter, the important thing is the process of writing and emotional release. Practice visualization of forgiveness, imagining yourself forgiving with love and compassion.

Forgiveness is a gift you give yourself, an act of liberation and healing. By forgiving, you free yourself from the past and make way for a lighter, happier, and more abundant future.

Chapter 16
Cultivating Abundance

In the previous chapters, we learned to free the heart from the weight of the past through forgiveness. Now, let's make room for gratitude, a powerful force that nourishes the soul and paves the way for abundance in all areas of life.

Imagine gratitude as a magnet that attracts into your life everything you appreciate and value. By cultivating gratitude, you shift the focus of your attention from what is lacking to what you already have, creating a virtuous cycle of positivity, joy, and abundance.

Gratitude is an emotion that arises when we recognize the value of something or someone in our lives. It is a feeling of appreciation, recognition, and contentment for the blessings we receive, big or small.

When we cultivate gratitude, we open our hearts to the abundance of the universe, recognizing the wealth that already exists in our lives and attracting even more prosperity, health, love, and happiness.

Opening your heart to gratitude:
- **Keep a gratitude journal:** Take time each day to write down in a journal the things you are grateful for. These can be simple things, like a sunny day,

a hug from a friend, a tasty meal, or a moment of inner peace.
- **Express your gratitude:** Thank the people in your life, express your appreciation for their qualities and for all they do for you.
- **Give thanks for the little things:** Cultivate gratitude for the little things in everyday life, such as a smile, a gesture of kindness, or a moment of beauty.
- **Connect with nature:** Spend time in contact with nature, appreciating the beauty of plants, animals, and the universe.
- **Practice gratitude meditation:** Find a quiet place, close your eyes, and focus on feelings of gratitude. Imagine all the good things you have in your life and feel the emotion of gratitude filling your heart.
- **Create a gratitude altar:** Create a space in your home dedicated to gratitude, where you can place objects that remind you of the things you are grateful for.
- **Celebrate your achievements:** Acknowledge and celebrate your achievements, big or small, and be grateful for the opportunities that led you to them.

The benefits of gratitude:
- **Increased happiness and well-being:** Gratitude increases the production of well-being hormones, such as serotonin and dopamine, promoting happiness, joy, and optimism.

- **Improved relationships:** Gratitude strengthens bonds and promotes connection with others.
- **Increased self-esteem:** Gratitude increases self-confidence and self-acceptance.
- **Reduced stress and anxiety:** Gratitude calms the mind and reduces the production of stress hormones.
- **Improved physical health:** Gratitude strengthens the immune system and promotes physical health.
- **Attracting abundance:** Gratitude creates a virtuous cycle of positivity and attracts prosperity, health, love, and happiness.

Exercise:

Start practicing gratitude today. Write down in a journal three things you are grateful for. Express your gratitude to someone you love. Connect with nature and give thanks for the beauty of the world around you.

Gratitude is a key that opens the doors to abundance in all areas of your life. By cultivating gratitude, you transform your reality, attracting more prosperity, health, love, and happiness.

Chapter 17
Ho'oponopono

In the previous chapters, we explored the power of gratitude to attract abundance. Now, let's delve into the profound Hawaiian wisdom of Ho'oponopono, a practice of healing and reconciliation that invites us to take responsibility for our reality and promote inner peace.

Imagine that everything you experience in your life, from the most pleasant events to the most difficult challenges, are reflections of your inner world. Ho'oponopono teaches us that we are 100% responsible for everything that happens in our lives, because everything we perceive in the outside world is a projection of what we carry within us.

This ancient practice is based on the belief that negative memories and beliefs stored in our subconscious create energy blocks that manifest as problems and conflicts in our lives. Ho'oponopono offers us a way to clear these memories, purify our minds, and restore inner harmony.

Through the repetition of four simple phrases – "I'm sorry," "Please forgive me," "Thank you," and "I love you" – we connect with the Divine and ask for the purification of our memories and limiting beliefs. By taking responsibility for our reality and asking for forgiveness, we open space for healing, reconciliation, and transformation.

The principles of Ho'oponopono:
- **Responsibility:** Take responsibility for everything that happens in your life, recognizing that your thoughts, feelings, and actions create your reality.
- **Forgiveness:** Ask forgiveness of yourself and others for any negative memory or belief that has contributed to the creation of problems and conflicts.
- **Love:** Cultivate unconditional love for yourself, others, and all forms of life.
- **Gratitude:** Give thanks for the blessings you already have and for all opportunities for growth and learning.

Applying Ho'oponopono:
- **Identify the problem:** When faced with a problem or conflict, recognize that it is a reflection of something that needs to be healed within you.
- **Repeat the four phrases:** Repeat mentally or aloud the phrases "I'm sorry," "Please forgive me," "Thank you," and "I love you," directing them to the situation or person involved.
- **Focus on purification:** Visualize the situation being purified by divine light, releasing the negative memories and beliefs that sustain it.
- **Practice consistently:** Ho'oponopono is a daily practice that requires consistency and dedication.

The more you practice, the deeper the healing and transformation in your life will be.

The benefits of Ho'oponopono:
- **Emotional healing:** Releases hurts, resentments, and traumas from the past.
- **Inner peace:** Promotes serenity, harmony, and emotional balance.
- **Improved relationships:** Restores relationships and promotes reconciliation.
- **Increased self-awareness:** Increases understanding of yourself and your patterns of thought and behavior.
- **Manifestation of desires:** Clears blocks that prevent the realization of your dreams and goals.
- **Spiritual connection:** Strengthens the connection with the Divine and promotes spiritual growth.

Exercise:

Choose a situation or person that causes you discomfort or conflict. Practice Ho'oponopono by repeating the four phrases sincerely and visualizing the situation being purified. Observe the changes that occur in your feelings and thoughts.

Ho'oponopono is a path of healing and transformation that invites you to take responsibility for your reality and promote inner peace. By clearing your memories and limiting beliefs, you open space for abundance, harmony, and happiness in your life.

Chapter 18
Balancing Vital Energy

In the previous chapters, we immersed ourselves in the wisdom of Ho'oponopono and learned to take responsibility for our reality. Now, let's explore Reiki, an energy healing technique that promotes balance and harmony through the gentle touch of hands.

Imagine vital energy as a river flowing through your body, nourishing every cell and organ. Reiki acts as a channel for this universal energy, allowing it to flow freely, removing blockages and restoring the body's natural balance.

Reiki is a Japanese healing technique that uses the laying on of hands to transmit vital energy. The word "Reiki" means "universal life energy," and this energy is channeled by the Reiki practitioner to the recipient, promoting relaxation, stress relief, and physical, emotional, and spiritual healing.

During a Reiki session, the practitioner gently places their hands on or near the recipient's body, at specific points called chakras, which are centers of vital energy. Reiki energy flows through the practitioner's hands, harmonizing the chakras, dissolving energy blocks, and promoting well-being.

The principles of Reiki:
- **Just for today, do not worry:** Free yourself from worries and live in the present moment with serenity.
- **Just for today, do not anger:** Cultivate patience, understanding, and compassion.
- **Honor your parents, teachers, and elders:** Show respect and gratitude for those who guide and inspire you.
- **Earn your living honestly:** Live with integrity, ethics, and honesty.
- **Show gratitude to all living beings:** Recognize the interconnectedness of all life forms and cultivate gratitude for existence.

The benefits of Reiki:
- **Deep relaxation:** Promotes physical and mental relaxation, relieving stress and anxiety.
- **Pain relief:** Helps relieve chronic and acute pain, promoting physical well-being.
- **Emotional balance:** Harmonizes emotions, reducing anxiety, depression, and other emotional imbalances.
- **Increased vital energy:** Revitalizes the body, increases vitality, and promotes health.
- **Acceleration of the healing process:** Strengthens the immune system and accelerates the body's natural healing process.
- **Spiritual development:** Promotes self-knowledge, spiritual connection, and personal growth.

Exercise:

Try a Reiki session with a qualified practitioner. Feel the Reiki energy flowing through your body, promoting relaxation, balance, and healing. Observe the sensations and emotions that arise during the session.

Reiki is a gift of healing and harmonization that invites you to connect with universal life energy. By receiving Reiki, you pave the way for physical, emotional, and spiritual well-being, and awaken your potential for healing and transformation.

Chapter 19
The Power of Stones in Holistic Healing

In the previous chapters, we explored universal vital energy through Reiki. Now, let's enter the mineral kingdom and discover the subtle yet profound power of Crystal Therapy, an ancient practice that uses the energetic vibrations of crystals to promote balance, healing, and well-being.

Imagine crystals as ancestral libraries of energy, each vibrating at a unique frequency, storing the wisdom of the Earth and emanating healing vibrations. Crystal Therapy is based on the belief that these vibrations interact with the human energy field, promoting the harmonization of the chakras, the dissolution of blockages, and the alignment of body, mind, and spirit.

Crystals are formed over millions of years in the heart of the Earth, absorbing energies and information from the environment around them. Each crystal has a unique molecular structure that determines its energetic and therapeutic properties. Crystal therapy uses this energy to promote physical, emotional, and spiritual well-being.

Understanding Crystal Therapy:
- **Each crystal has a unique vibration:** Just as each person has a unique fingerprint, each crystal

vibrates at a specific frequency, with distinct healing and energetic properties.
- **Crystals interact with the human energy field:** Upon contact with the human body, crystals interact with the energy field, promoting balance and harmonization.
- **The choice of crystal is intuitive and personal:** Choosing the ideal crystal for each person or situation can be done intuitively, feeling the energy of the stone and connecting with its vibration.
- **Crystals can be used in a variety of ways:** Crystals can be used during meditation, placed on the body, worn as jewelry, carried in your pocket, or used in environments to harmonize energy.

Some crystals and their properties:
- **Clear Quartz:** Amplifies energy, promotes mental clarity and healing.
- **Amethyst:** Calms the mind, transmutes negative energies and promotes intuition.
- **Rose Quartz:** Opens the heart to love, compassion and emotional healing.
- **Citrine:** Attracts prosperity, abundance and joy.
- **Selenite:** Purifies energy, promotes inner peace and spiritual connection.
- **Tiger's Eye:** Protects against negative energies, increases self-confidence and inner strength.

The benefits of Crystal Therapy:
- **Energy balance:** Harmonizes the chakras and promotes the free flow of vital energy.

- **Physical healing:** Helps relieve pain, inflammation and other physical imbalances.
- **Emotional healing:** Releases negative emotions, traumas and emotional blocks.
- **Inner peace:** Promotes serenity, harmony and mental well-being.
- **Increased intuition:** Awakens intuition, creativity and spiritual connection.
- **Energy protection:** Creates a protective shield against negative energies and external influences.

Exercise:

Choose a crystal that catches your eye and hold it in your hands. Feel its energy, its temperature, its texture. Allow your intuition to guide you in choosing the ideal crystal for you. Use the crystal during meditation, carry it with you or place it in an environment you wish to harmonize.

Crystals are powerful allies on the journey of self-knowledge and healing. By connecting with the energy of crystals, you awaken the power of inner healing and open the way to balance, harmony and transformation.

Chapter 20
Values and Life Purposes

In the previous chapters, we explored the power of crystals in holistic healing. Now, let's embark on an even deeper journey of self-discovery, seeking to unravel your values and life purposes, the compass that guides your choices and propels you towards personal fulfillment.

Imagine life as a great journey, with various possible paths and destinations. Your values and purposes are like a map that guides you on this journey, helping you choose the paths that will lead you to the destinations that really matter to you.

Values are principles that guide your decisions and actions, what you consider important and meaningful in your life. Purposes, in turn, are your life goals, what motivates you to move forward and gives you the feeling that your life has meaning.

Discovering your values and purpose is like finding a hidden treasure within yourself. It is connecting with your essence, with your soul, and discovering what truly makes you vibrate, what inspires you and what drives you to be your best version.

Exploring your values and purposes:
- **Reflect on your experiences:** What were the most significant experiences of your life? What did you learn from them? What values did they reveal about you?
- **Identify your talents and passions:** What do you do with ease and pleasure? What are your natural abilities? What excites and motivates you?
- **Imagine your ideal future:** How do you see yourself in 5, 10 or 20 years? What will you be doing? What will your accomplishments be? How will you feel?
- **Connect with your intuition:** Pay attention to your feelings and intuitions. What does your heart tell you about your values and purpose?
- **Try new things:** Explore different areas of interest, participate in activities that challenge and inspire you. Experimentation helps you discover new talents and passions.
- **Seek inspiration:** Talk to people you admire, read books and watch movies that inspire you. Inspiration helps you connect with your values and purpose.
- **Define your values:** Create a list of the values that are most important to you, such as honesty, compassion, freedom, creativity, justice, etc.
- **Write your purpose statement:** Write a statement that expresses your life goals, what motivates you to move forward and gives you the feeling that your life has meaning.

The benefits of knowing your values and purpose:
- **Clarity and direction:** Helps you make decisions that are more aligned with your values and goals.
- **Motivation and purpose:** Drives you to move forward and pursue your dreams.
- **Personal fulfillment:** Leads you to a more authentic, meaningful and fulfilling life.
- **Self-knowledge:** Helps you connect with your essence and discover who you really are.
- **Emotional well-being:** Promotes inner peace, happiness and personal satisfaction.

Exercise:

Take some time to reflect on the questions above. Write down your answers in a journal and review them periodically. Create your list of values and write your purpose statement.

Your values and purpose are like a beacon that illuminates your path and guides you towards personal fulfillment. By discovering and living them, you transform your life into a journey of meaning, purpose and happiness.

Chapter 21
Unleashing Your Unique Potential

In the previous chapter, we began the journey of self-discovery by exploring your values and life purpose. Now, let's delve deeper into discovering your talents and abilities, the inner resources that make you unique and empower you to achieve your dreams.

Imagine a chest full of precious jewels, each with its own unique brilliance and value. Your talents and abilities are like these jewels, gifts that you bring with you and that can be polished and used to create a full and meaningful life.

Talents are natural aptitudes, innate abilities that you have to perform certain activities with ease and excellence. Skills, in turn, are abilities developed through practice and learning, which allow you to perform tasks and achieve specific goals.

Discovering your talents and abilities is like unraveling a map that guides you towards your maximum potential. It is recognizing your gifts, your passions and your areas of excellence, and using them to create an authentic, prosperous and fulfilling life.

Exploring your talents and abilities:
- **Observe what you do with ease:** What activities do you perform naturally and with pleasure, effortlessly? What flows naturally to you?
- **Identify your strengths:** What are your most striking characteristics? What do people compliment you on? What are your areas of excellence?
- **Pay attention to your interests:** What fascinates and attracts you? What subjects arouse your curiosity and desire to learn?
- **Recall your experiences:** What were your greatest successes and achievements? What activities gave you the most satisfaction and fulfillment?
- **Try new things:** Explore different areas of knowledge, participate in courses and workshops, practice activities that challenge and inspire you.
- **Ask for feedback:** Talk to people who know you well and ask for feedback on your talents and abilities.
- **Take vocational tests:** Use vocational tests to identify your areas of aptitude and interest.
- **Write down your findings:** Keep a journal to record your talents, skills, interests and passions.

The benefits of knowing your talents and abilities:
- **Self-knowledge:** Increases understanding of yourself, your capabilities and your unique potential.

- **Self-confidence:** Strengthens belief in yourself and your abilities.
- **Motivation:** Drives you to pursue your dreams and goals with more confidence and determination.
- **Professional achievement:** Helps you choose a career that is aligned with your talents and passions.
- **Personal growth:** Encourages you to develop your skills and seek your full potential.
- **Creativity:** Stimulates the expression of your creativity and the search for new ways to use your talents.

Exercise:

Make a list of your talents and abilities. Recall your experiences and identify the activities that gave you the most satisfaction and fulfillment. Ask for feedback from people who know you well. Explore new areas of knowledge and try new things.

Your talents and abilities are gifts you have received to share with the world. By recognizing and utilizing them, you contribute to building a more authentic, prosperous and meaningful life, both for yourself and for those around you.

Chapter 22
Breaking Free from the Chains of Thought

In previous chapters, we uncovered your values, purpose, talents and abilities, revealing a map to your unique potential. Now, let's break free from the chains that can prevent you from reaching that potential: limiting beliefs.

Imagine the mind as a fertile garden, ready to bloom. Limiting beliefs are like weeds that suck nutrients from the soil, preventing the full growth of your potential. They are negative and distorted thoughts about yourself, the world and the future, which imprison you in cycles of fear, insecurity and self-sabotage.

These beliefs can have deep roots, originating in past experiences, negative messages received in childhood, or dysfunctional thought patterns. They disguise themselves as "absolute truths", whispering phrases in your ear like "I am not capable", "I don't deserve", "I always fail" or "This is impossible for me".

Overcoming limiting beliefs is like pulling these weeds out by the roots, freeing the soil of your mind so that your dreams can flourish. It is a process of self-knowledge, questioning and transformation, which empowers you to rewrite your story and create a more positive and abundant reality.

Identifying and transforming limiting beliefs:
- **Be aware of your thoughts:** Notice the thoughts that arise in your mind, especially those that cause you fear, anxiety or insecurity.
- **Identify the beliefs behind the thoughts:** What are the "truths" that support these thoughts? What messages have you received throughout your life that reinforce these beliefs?
- **Question the validity of beliefs:** Are they really true? Is there evidence to support them? What are the other possible perspectives?
- **Rewrite beliefs:** Replace limiting beliefs with positive and empowering affirmations. Instead of "I am not capable", affirm "I am capable of achieving my dreams".
- **Seek evidence that contradicts beliefs:** Recall your successes, your achievements and the times you overcame challenges.
- **Visualize yourself overcoming beliefs:** Imagine yourself acting with confidence, courage and determination, free from the shackles of limiting beliefs.
- **Surround yourself with positive people:** Connect with people who support you, inspire you and encourage you to grow.
- **Seek professional help:** If necessary, seek the help of a therapist or coach to assist you in this transformation process.

The benefits of overcoming limiting beliefs:
- **Emotional freedom:** Free yourself from fear, insecurity and self-sabotage.

- **Self-confidence:** Increase belief in yourself and your abilities.
- **Goal achievement:** Achieve your dreams and live a fuller and more authentic life.
- **Improved relationships:** Build healthier and more authentic relationships.
- **Personal growth:** Expand your horizons and explore your full potential.

Exercise:

Identify a limiting belief that is preventing you from achieving your goals. Question its validity, look for evidence that contradicts it, and rewrite it in a positive and empowering way. Visualize yourself overcoming this belief and acting with confidence and determination.

You are much more powerful than you think. By freeing yourself from limiting beliefs, you open the way to a life of infinite possibilities, where your dreams come true and your potential flourishes in its fullness.

Chapter 23
Self-Esteem and Self-Confidence

In the previous chapters, we removed the weeds of limiting beliefs from the garden of your mind. Now, it's time to nurture the fertile soil of your self-esteem and self-confidence, the pillars that support personal growth and the achievement of your dreams.

Imagine self-esteem as the deep roots of a majestic tree, which nourish and sustain it, allowing it to grow strong and imposing. Self-confidence, in turn, is the branches that extend towards the sky, seeking light and expansion.

Self-esteem is the value you place on yourself, how you see and feel about yourself. It is the foundation of your identity, the belief in your intrinsic worth, regardless of your achievements or the approval of others.

Self-confidence, on the other hand, is the belief in your abilities, the certainty that you can achieve your goals and overcome challenges. It is the inner strength that drives you to act, to take risks and to pursue your dreams.

Developing self-esteem and self-confidence is like building a solid foundation for your personal growth. It is nurturing your essence, recognizing your qualities, accepting your imperfections and believing in your infinite potential.

Cultivating self-esteem and self-confidence:
- **Recognize your qualities:** Make a list of your qualities, talents, skills and achievements. Celebrate your successes and recognize your intrinsic worth.
- **Accept your imperfections:** Be kind to yourself, recognizing that we all have flaws and imperfections. Accept yourself as you are, with love and compassion.
- **Practice self-compassion:** Treat yourself with the same kindness and understanding that you would treat a dear friend. Forgive yourself for your mistakes and celebrate your progress.
- **Affirm your worth:** Repeat positive affirmations that reinforce your self-esteem and self-confidence, such as "I am worthy of love", "I am capable" and "I deserve the best".
- **Take care of yourself:** Prioritize your physical and mental health by eating well, exercising, getting enough sleep and making time for activities that bring you pleasure and relaxation.
- **Set realistic goals:** Set challenging but achievable goals, and celebrate each achievement along the way.
- **Learn from your mistakes:** See mistakes as opportunities for learning and growth, instead of blaming or criticizing yourself.
- **Surround yourself with positive people:** Cultivate relationships with people who support

you, inspire you and encourage you to be your best version.
- **Seek professional help:** If necessary, seek the help of a therapist or coach to assist you in this process of personal development.

The benefits of self-esteem and self-confidence:
- **Emotional well-being:** Increases happiness, resilience and the ability to deal with challenges.
- **Personal fulfillment:** Drives you to pursue your dreams and achieve your goals.
- **Improved relationships:** Promotes healthier and more authentic relationships.
- **Professional success:** Increases productivity, creativity and leadership skills.
- **Physical health:** Strengthens the immune system and promotes physical health.

Exercise:

Write a love letter to yourself, recognizing your qualities, accepting your imperfections and expressing your gratitude for who you are. Repeat positive affirmations that reinforce your self-esteem and self-confidence.

You are a unique and special person, with qualities and talents that make you amazing. By cultivating self-esteem and self-confidence, you nurture your essence, strengthen your roots and allow yourself to flourish in your fullness.

Chapter 24
Assertive Communication

In the previous chapters, we strengthened the foundation of your personal growth by cultivating self-esteem and self-confidence. Now, let's build bridges to the outside world, learning to communicate your needs clearly, respectfully and authentically, through assertive communication.

Imagine communication as a dance, where each person expresses their movements and connects with the other in harmony. Assertive communication is like a fluid and balanced dance, where you express your ideas, feelings and needs with clarity and respect, while listening and considering the other.

Being assertive is like finding the balance point between passivity, which leads you to silence your needs and nullify yourself, and aggressiveness, which leads you to impose your will and disrespect the other. It is communicating directly, honestly and respectfully, defending your rights and expressing your opinions without attacking or submitting.

Assertive communication is an essential skill for building healthy relationships, resolving conflicts constructively and achieving your goals effectively. It is the key to expressing your truth, setting boundaries and creating authentic connections with the people around you.

Developing assertive communication:

- **Connect with your needs:** Identify your needs, desires and feelings before communicating. What do you really want to express? What do you need from the other person?
- **Express yourself clearly and objectively:** Communicate your ideas clearly, concisely and directly, using clear and objective language.
- **Use body language:** Maintain an upright posture, eye contact and a firm and calm tone of voice. Your body language should convey confidence and respect.
- **Listen actively:** Pay attention to what the other person is saying, showing interest and empathy. Ask questions to clarify doubts and show that you are really listening.
- **Express your feelings:** Communicate your feelings authentically and respectfully, using phrases like "I feel..." or "I need...".
- **Set boundaries:** Communicate your boundaries clearly and firmly, saying "no" when necessary and expressing your expectations clearly.
- **Seek solutions together:** In conflict situations, seek solutions that meet the needs of both parties, using negotiation and collaboration.
- **Practice empathy:** Try to put yourself in the other person's shoes, understanding their feelings and perspectives.

- **Be patient and persistent:** Developing assertive communication takes time and practice. Be patient with yourself and persist in your efforts.

The benefits of assertive communication:
- **Improved relationships:** Build healthier, more authentic and satisfying relationships.
- **Conflict reduction:** Resolve conflicts constructively and peacefully.
- **Increased self-esteem:** Strengthens self-confidence and self-respect.
- **Personal fulfillment:** Achieve your goals and express your truth authentically.
- **Emotional well-being:** Reduces stress, anxiety and frustration.

Exercise:

Identify a situation where you had difficulty communicating assertively. Reflect on how you could have expressed yourself more clearly, respectfully and authentically. Practice assertive communication in everyday situations, expressing your needs and setting boundaries.

Assertive communication is a powerful tool for building bridges, expressing your truth and creating authentic connections with the world around you. By mastering this skill, you become a more effective, confident and authentic communicator.

Chapter 25
Authentic and Nourishing Connections

In the previous chapters, we learned to communicate our needs assertively, building bridges to the outside world. Now, let's delve into the art of creating healthy relationships, cultivating authentic and nourishing connections that enrich our lives and propel us towards well-being and happiness.

Imagine relationships as a garden, where each person is a unique flower, with its colors, shapes and scents. Creating healthy relationships is like tending this garden with care and attention, nurturing each flower so that it blooms in its fullness, contributing to the beauty and harmony of the whole.

Healthy relationships are like fertile ground where love, respect, trust and reciprocity flourish. They are connections that nourish the soul, inspire growth and drive us to be our best versions.

Building healthy relationships requires self-knowledge, assertive communication, empathy and compassion. It is a process of constant learning, which involves the ability to connect with the other authentically, respecting their individuality and cultivating reciprocity.

Cultivating healthy relationships:
- **Cultivate self-love:** The basis for building healthy relationships is self-love. Recognize your worth, take care of yourself and treat yourself with kindness and respect.
- **Be authentic:** Show yourself as you truly are, without masks or disguises. Share your thoughts, feelings and dreams with the people you love.
- **Communicate openly:** Express your needs, desires and boundaries clearly and respectfully. Listen carefully to what the other person has to say, showing interest and empathy.
- **Cultivate respect:** Respect the differences, opinions and boundaries of the other. Value the individuality of each person and recognize their intrinsic worth.
- **Practice empathy:** Try to put yourself in the other person's shoes, understanding their feelings and perspectives. Show compassion and support in difficult times.
- **Spend quality time:** Set aside time to be present with the people you love, sharing special moments and creating emotional memories.
- **Cultivate reciprocity:** Offer support, affection and attention, and be willing to receive the same in return. Healthy relationships are based on reciprocity and balance.
- **Set healthy boundaries:** Communicate your boundaries clearly and respectfully, protecting your energy and well-being.

- **Learn to forgive:** Forgive yourself and others, releasing hurt and resentment that can harm the relationship.
- **Celebrate differences:** Recognize that each person is unique and special, and celebrate the differences that enrich the relationship.

The benefits of healthy relationships:
- **Emotional well-being:** Increases happiness, self-esteem and sense of belonging.
- **Emotional support:** Offers support, comfort and security in difficult times.
- **Personal growth:** Inspires growth, evolution and the pursuit of self-knowledge.
- **Physical health:** Strengthens the immune system and promotes physical health.
- **Longevity:** People with healthy relationships tend to live longer and with a better quality of life.

Exercise:

Reflect on the relationships in your life. Which relationships nurture and inspire you? Which relationships need to be cultivated or transformed? Communicate your needs and expectations assertively, seeking to build more authentic and nourishing connections.

Healthy relationships are like a flowering garden, which requires care, attention and dedication. By cultivating authentic and nourishing connections, you enrich your life, strengthen your soul and open yourself to love, happiness and fulfillment.

Chapter 26
Goals and Objectives

In the previous chapters, we learned to cultivate healthy relationships, creating authentic connections that nurture and propel us. Now, let's turn our focus to the future, learning to define goals and objectives that guide us towards the realization of our dreams and aspirations.

Imagine life as a ship sailing the high seas. Goals and objectives are like the map and compass that guide the ship, setting the course and directing it to the desired destination. Without a map and compass, the ship is adrift, subject to the whims of the wind and sea currents.

Setting goals is like drawing up a plan for your life, establishing clear and specific objectives that motivate you to move forward and give you a sense of purpose and direction. It is like building a detailed map, with each step defined, each obstacle anticipated and each achievement celebrated.

Well-defined goals drive you to get out of your comfort zone, overcome challenges and achieve extraordinary results. They help you focus your energy, organize your time and use your resources efficiently, turning your dreams into reality.

Defining effective goals:
- **Dream big:** Start by visualizing your dreams and aspirations, without being limited by limiting beliefs or fears. What do you really want to achieve in your life?
- **Be specific:** Define your goals clearly, specifically and measurably. Instead of "I want to be rich", define "I want to have a monthly income of X dollars".
- **Set deadlines:** Set realistic deadlines to achieve your goals, breaking them down into smaller steps and setting short, medium and long-term goals.
- **Create an action plan:** Define the actions needed to achieve your goals, step by step. What resources do you need? What skills do you need to develop? What obstacles do you need to overcome?
- **Stay focused:** Focus your energy and efforts on achieving your goals, avoiding distractions and maintaining discipline.
- **Monitor your progress:** Track your progress regularly, evaluating your results and adjusting your action plan when necessary.
- **Celebrate your achievements:** Recognize and celebrate each achievement along the way, no matter how small. Celebration motivates you to keep going and drives you towards success.
- **Be flexible:** Be open to adjusting your goals and plans when necessary, adapting to changes and learning from experiences.

- **Visualize your goals:** Use creative visualization to imagine your goals as if they were already real, feeling the emotions and sensations of having already achieved them.
- **Believe in yourself:** Trust in your ability to achieve your dreams and maintain a positive and persevering attitude.

The benefits of setting goals:
- **Direction and purpose:** Gives you clarity about your goals and drives you towards achieving your dreams.
- **Motivation and focus:** Increases your motivation, helps you focus your efforts and avoid distractions.
- **Organization and planning:** Helps you organize your time, resources and actions efficiently.
- **Productivity and efficiency:** Increases your productivity and helps you achieve extraordinary results.
- **Self-knowledge:** Helps you understand your values, priorities and dreams.
- **Personal fulfillment:** Leads you to a fuller, more meaningful and fulfilling life.

Exercise:

Define three goals that you want to achieve in the next few months. Be specific, measurable, achievable, relevant and time-bound. Create a detailed action plan, with the steps needed to achieve each goal. Visualize your goals as if they were already real and celebrate each achievement along the way.

Setting goals is like drawing a map to success, guiding you towards the realization of your dreams and aspirations. By setting clear, specific and challenging goals, you empower yourself to create the life you want and live with purpose, passion and fulfillment.

Chapter 27
Organizing Your Actions and Resources

In the previous chapter, we learned how to define goals and objectives, drawing the map to achieve your dreams. Now, let's build the vehicle that will take you to that destination: planning.

Imagine planning as the construction of a robust and well-equipped ship, capable of navigating the seas of life with safety and efficiency. Each piece, each tool, each carefully planned detail contributes to the solidity of the vessel and increases the chances of reaching the desired destination.

Planning is the art of organizing your actions, your resources, and your time strategically, aiming to achieve your goals effectively. It's like building a bridge that connects the present to the future, turning your dreams into reality.

Good planning helps you define priorities, avoid distractions, overcome obstacles, and use your resources intelligently. It gives you clarity, organization, and control over your life, increasing your chances of success in all areas.

Building an effective plan:
- **Define your objectives:** Start by reviewing your goals and objectives, ensuring they are clear, specific, and measurable.
- **Divide into stages:** Break your goals into smaller, more manageable steps, setting short, medium, and long-term goals.
- **Identify your resources:** What resources do you have to achieve your goals? Consider your talents, skills, time, money, contacts, and other available resources.
- **Create a schedule:** Establish a realistic schedule for each stage of your plan, setting deadlines for each task.
- **Organize your tasks:** Use organizational tools, such as calendars, to-do lists, apps, or time management software to organize your tasks and priorities.
- **Define priorities:** Identify the most important and urgent tasks, focusing your efforts on those that will get you closer to your goals.
- **Anticipate obstacles:** What are the possible obstacles you may encounter along the way? How can you prepare to overcome them?
- **Be flexible:** Be open to adjusting your plan when necessary, adapting to changes and learning from experiences.
- **Monitor your progress:** Track your progress regularly, evaluating your results and adjusting your action plan when necessary.

- **Celebrate your achievements:** Acknowledge and celebrate each achievement along the way, no matter how small. Celebration motivates you to move forward and propels you toward success.

The benefits of planning:
- **Organization and efficiency:** Increases your organization, helps you manage your time and resources efficiently.
- **Clarity and focus:** Gives you clarity about your goals and helps you stay focused on your priorities.
- **Stress reduction:** Reduces stress and anxiety, providing a sense of control over your life.
- **Increased productivity:** Increases your productivity, helping you accomplish more in less time.
- **Improved decision making:** Helps you make more strategic and effective decisions.
- **Achievement of goals:** Increases your chances of achieving your goals and fulfilling your dreams.

Exercise:

Choose a goal you want to achieve and create a detailed plan to achieve it. Define the steps, deadlines, necessary resources, and possible obstacles. Use organizational tools to manage your tasks and monitor your progress regularly.

Planning is the compass that guides you towards success, turning your dreams into reality. By planning your actions, your resources, and your time strategically, you empower yourself to create the life you want and live with purpose, passion, and fulfillment.

Chapter 28
Procrastination

In the previous chapters, we learned how to plan for success by strategically organizing our actions and resources. Now, let's face one of the biggest obstacles that can prevent us from achieving our goals: procrastination.

Imagine procrastination as a weight that holds you to the ground, preventing you from flying towards your dreams. It is the art of postponing tasks, finding excuses, and getting distracted by less important activities while responsibilities and goals take a back seat.

Procrastination is like a trap that deceives you with the promise of immediate pleasure while taking you away from fulfilling your dreams and leading you to a cycle of frustration, guilt, and anxiety. It manifests itself in different ways, from the classic "leaving it for later" to the more subtle "paralyzing perfectionism."

Overcoming procrastination is like freeing yourself from this weight, spreading your wings, and flying towards your goals. It is taking control of your time, your actions, and your life, transforming inertia into action and procrastination into productivity.

Overcoming procrastination:
- **Identify the causes:** Why do you procrastinate? What are the fears, limiting beliefs, or difficulties that prevent you from taking action?
- **Set clear and realistic goals:** Vague or complex goals can be intimidating and lead you to procrastinate. Set clear, specific, and realistic goals, breaking them down into smaller, more manageable steps.
- **Prioritize your tasks:** Use organizational tools, such as to-do lists or Eisenhower matrices, to prioritize your tasks and focus on the most important and urgent ones.
- **Eliminate distractions:** Create a distraction-free work environment by turning off your cell phone, notifications, and social media while you focus on your tasks.
- **Break tasks into small parts:** Large and complex tasks can be paralyzing. Break them down into smaller parts, making them easier to accomplish.
- **Start with the easiest:** If you feel unmotivated, start with an easier and more enjoyable task to gain momentum and enter a state of flow.
- **Use the Pomodoro Technique:** This technique consists of working in 25-minute time blocks with short 5-minute breaks between each block.
- **Reward yourself for achievements:** Celebrate each completed task by rewarding yourself with something that motivates you and gives you pleasure.

- **Practice self-compassion:** Don't blame or criticize yourself for procrastinating. Acknowledge that we all procrastinate at some point and focus on learning from your mistakes and moving on.
- **Seek support:** Share your goals and challenges with friends, family, or a coach, seeking support and motivation to overcome procrastination.

The benefits of overcoming procrastination:
- **Increased productivity:** Accomplish more in less time, achieving your goals more efficiently.
- **Stress reduction:** Reduce stress and anxiety by eliminating feelings of overload and guilt.
- **Improved self-esteem:** Increase your self-esteem and self-confidence by feeling capable of completing your tasks and achieving your goals.
- **Personal fulfillment:** Achieve your dreams and live a fuller and more authentic life.
- **Freedom and empowerment:** Take control of your time, your actions, and your life.

Exercise:

Identify a task you are procrastinating on. Analyze the causes of procrastination and define strategies to overcome it. Break the task into small parts, eliminate distractions, and use the Pomodoro Technique to stay focused. Celebrate each completed step and reward yourself for your progress.

Procrastination is a habit that can be overcome with self-awareness, discipline, and persistence. By overcoming procrastination, you free yourself from the shackles of inertia and take control of your life, making your dreams a reality.

Chapter 29
The Art of Persistence

In the previous chapters, we learned how to plan for success and overcome procrastination. Now, let's strengthen the muscles of discipline and focus, the essential tools to turn your plans into reality and achieve your goals with mastery.

Imagine discipline as a steady rudder that guides the ship through storms and rough seas. It is the inner strength that keeps you on course, drives you to move forward even in the face of difficulties, and helps you resist temptations and distractions.

Focus, in turn, is the sail that propels the ship, capturing the energy of the wind and directing it towards the desired destination. It is the ability to focus your attention on what really matters, eliminating distractions and directing all your energy towards achieving your goals.

Cultivating discipline and focus is like training an athlete for a marathon. It requires effort, dedication, and persistence, but the reward is reaching the finish line, fulfilling your dreams, and exceeding your limits.

Mastering the art of discipline and focus:
- **Set clear and inspiring goals:** Clear and inspiring goals motivate you to stay disciplined

and focused, giving you a sense of purpose and direction.
- **Create a routine:** Establish a daily routine that includes time for your important activities, such as work, studies, exercise, and moments of relaxation.
- **Eliminate distractions:** Identify and eliminate distractions that prevent you from concentrating, such as cell phone notifications, social media, and unnecessary interruptions.
- **Practice mindfulness:** Cultivate mindfulness in your daily life by observing your thoughts and emotions without judgment and bringing your attention back to the present moment.
- **Use time management techniques:** Try techniques such as the Pomodoro Technique, which divides time into blocks of work and rest, to increase your productivity and focus.
- **Set priorities:** Prioritize your tasks, focusing on those that are most important and urgent to achieve your goals.
- **Learn to say "no":** Say "no" to activities and commitments that deviate you from your goals and disperse your energy.
- **Cultivate persistence:** Stay firm in your purposes, even in the face of difficulties and challenges. Remember that persistence is the key to achieving success.
- **Reward yourself for your progress:** Celebrate every achievement, no matter how small, rewarding yourself for your effort and dedication.

- **Practice self-compassion:** Be kind to yourself in times of difficulty, recognizing that discipline and focus are skills that are developed with practice.

The benefits of discipline and focus:
- **Increased productivity:** Accomplish more in less time, achieving your goals more efficiently.
- **Achievement of goals:** Increases your chances of achieving your goals and fulfilling your dreams.
- **Improved self-esteem:** Strengthens self-confidence and the feeling of control over your life.
- **Stress reduction:** Reduces stress and anxiety, providing a sense of organization and control.
- **Personal growth:** Develops your capacity for persistence, resilience, and self-control.
- **Professional success:** Increases your chances of success in your career, making you a more efficient and focused professional.

Exercise:

Choose an area of your life where you want to have more discipline and focus. Set clear goals, create a routine, eliminate distractions, and use time management techniques. Practice mindfulness and persistence, celebrating every achievement along the way.

Discipline and focus are like muscles that are strengthened with training. By cultivating these skills, you become the master of your destiny, navigating with security and determination towards your goals and achieving success in all areas of your life.

Chapter 30
Resilience

In the previous chapters, we built a solid foundation for success by cultivating discipline and focus. Now, let's prepare to face the inevitable storms of life by developing resilience, the ability to adapt, overcome challenges, and emerge stronger in the face of adversity.

Imagine resilience as the strength of a bamboo that bends in the wind but does not break. It is the ability to adapt to changes, recover from difficulties, and use challenges as opportunities for growth and learning.

Life is a journey full of ups and downs, moments of joy and moments of challenge. Resilience is what allows us to navigate these turbulent seas with courage, flexibility, and optimism, turning obstacles into springboards for success.

Developing resilience is like building an inner fortress that protects you from adversity and drives you forward, even when the path becomes difficult. It is the art of turning difficulties into opportunities, learning from mistakes, and using challenging experiences as fuel for personal growth.

Strengthening your resilience:
- **Cultivate optimism:** Maintain a positive attitude in the face of challenges, seeking to see opportunities for learning and growth in every situation.
- **Develop self-confidence:** Believe in your ability to overcome obstacles and find creative solutions to problems.
- **Strengthen your relationships:** Cultivate healthy relationships with people who support you, inspire you, and encourage you to move forward.
- **Learn from your mistakes:** See mistakes as opportunities for learning and growth, rather than blaming or criticizing yourself.
- **Practice gratitude:** Focus on the good things in your life and be thankful for them, cultivating an attitude of positivity and hope.
- **Take care of your physical and mental health:** Eat well, exercise regularly, get enough sleep, and engage in activities that bring you pleasure and relaxation.
- **Develop problem-solving skills:** Learn to identify problems, analyze causes, and find creative and effective solutions.
- **Seek professional support:** If necessary, seek the help of a therapist or coach to help you develop your resilience and deal with challenging situations.
- **Accept changes:** Be open to changes and adapt to new situations with flexibility and positivity.

- **Cultivate persistence:** Stay firm in your purposes, even in the face of difficulties and challenges. Remember that persistence is the key to achieving success.

The benefits of resilience:
- **Overcoming challenges:** Empowers you to face and overcome adversity with more strength and courage.
- **Personal growth:** Transforms challenges into opportunities for learning and growth.
- **Emotional well-being:** Increases happiness, self-esteem, and the ability to deal with stress.
- **Mental health:** Reduces the risk of developing anxiety, depression, and other mental health problems.
- **Professional success:** Increases your chances of success in your career, making you a more adaptable and resilient professional.
- **Stronger relationships:** Strengthens your relationships, making you a more understanding and supportive person.

Exercise:

Reflect on a challenge you faced in the past. How did you deal with this situation? What did you learn from this experience? How can you use this experience to strengthen your resilience and prepare for future challenges?

Resilience is the inner strength that allows you to overcome life's storms and emerge stronger and wiser. By cultivating resilience, you become an experienced navigator, able to face challenges with courage, optimism, and determination, turning obstacles into opportunities and building a life of success and fulfillment.

Chapter 31
Emotional Intelligence

In the previous chapters, we learned how to navigate the storms of life with resilience. Now, let's delve into the universe of emotional intelligence, the compass that guides us in understanding and managing emotions, both our own and those of others, to build a more fulfilling, authentic, and happy life.

Imagine emotional intelligence as a set of tools that allows you to navigate the complex world of emotions with mastery. It is the ability to recognize, understand, manage, and use emotions intelligently, both in relation to yourself and in your relationships with others.

Emotional intelligence goes beyond Intelligence Quotient (IQ), which measures cognitive abilities. It encompasses the ability to connect with yourself, to relate to others with empathy, to deal with adversity with resilience, and to make conscious and balanced decisions.

Developing emotional intelligence is like learning to speak the language of emotions, understanding their nuances, their signals, and their messages. It is the key to building healthier relationships, achieving your goals more effectively, and living with more harmony, balance, and well-being.

Developing emotional intelligence in practice:
- **Emotional self-awareness:** Pay attention to your emotions, learn to identify them, name them, and understand their causes and consequences.
- **Emotional management:** Develop strategies to deal with challenging emotions, such as anger, fear, sadness, and frustration, in a healthy and constructive way.
- **Self-motivation:** Cultivate intrinsic motivation by finding purpose and meaning in your actions and propelling yourself toward your goals.
- **Empathy:** Develop the ability to put yourself in another person's shoes, understanding their feelings, perspectives, and needs.
- **Social skills:** Improve your communication skills by learning to express yourself clearly, assertively, and respectfully, to listen actively, and to build healthy interpersonal relationships.

Applying emotional intelligence in everyday life:
- **Communication:** Express your ideas and feelings clearly, assertively, and respectfully, using body language and active listening to build effective communication.
- **Relationships:** Cultivate healthy relationships based on respect, trust, empathy, and reciprocity. Learn to deal with conflict constructively and express your needs assertively.

- **Work:** Use emotional intelligence to increase your productivity, build a positive work environment, lead teams effectively, and achieve your professional goals.
- **Mental health:** Manage stress, anxiety, and other challenging emotions by cultivating self-awareness, resilience, and emotional well-being.
- **Decision making:** Make more conscious and balanced decisions, considering both rational and emotional aspects.

The benefits of emotional intelligence:
- **Emotional well-being:** Increases happiness, self-esteem, resilience, and the ability to cope with challenges.
- **Improved relationships:** Promotes healthier, more authentic, and satisfying relationships.
- **Professional success:** Increases productivity, creativity, and leadership ability.
- **Physical health:** Reduces stress, strengthens the immune system, and promotes physical health.
- **Personal fulfillment:** Leads you to a more fulfilling, authentic, and meaningful life.

Exercise:

Identify a situation where you could have used emotional intelligence more effectively. Reflect on how you can use the tools of emotional intelligence to communicate better, build healthier relationships, manage your emotions, and achieve your goals.

Emotional intelligence is a compass that guides you on the path of self-discovery, personal growth, and fulfillment. By developing this skill, you become the master of your emotions, building a more fulfilling, authentic, and happy life.

Chapter 32
Unraveling the Mind-Body Connection

In the previous chapters, we explored the power of emotional intelligence to navigate the waves of emotions. Now, let's dive into the fascinating mind-body connection, discovering how our thoughts, emotions, and beliefs can influence our physical health and well-being.

Imagine the mind and body as two sides of the same coin, interconnected and interdependent. The mind, with its thoughts, emotions, and beliefs, directly influences the body, impacting its functioning, its reactions, and its health.

This mind-body connection is a two-way street. Just as the mind influences the body, the body also sends signals to the mind, through sensations, pain, and other physical symptoms. Understanding this interaction is fundamental to taking care of health in an integral way and promoting well-being at all levels of being.

Modern science has increasingly proven the influence of the mind on the body. Studies show that chronic stress, anxiety, depression, and other negative emotions can weaken the immune system, increase the risk of heart disease, trigger chronic pain, and affect the functioning of various organs.

On the other hand, positive emotions, such as joy, gratitude, and optimism, strengthen the immune system, promote cardiovascular health, accelerate the healing process, and increase the feeling of well-being.

Unraveling the mind-body connection:
- **The power of thoughts:** Negative thoughts and limiting beliefs can generate stress, anxiety, and fear, negatively impacting physical health. Positive thoughts and empowering beliefs promote health, well-being, and healing.
- **The influence of emotions:** Emotions such as anger, sadness, and fear can trigger physiological reactions such as increased blood pressure, muscle tension, and the release of stress hormones. Positive emotions, such as joy, gratitude, and love, promote relaxation, well-being, and health.
- **The role of stress:** Chronic stress is one of the main factors contributing to the development of physical and mental illnesses. Learning to manage stress is fundamental to health and well-being.
- **The importance of self-care:** Taking care of physical and mental health is essential to maintain the balance of the mind-body connection. Healthy eating, physical exercise, restful sleep, relaxation, and self-awareness practices are pillars of self-care.
- **The power of visualization:** Creative visualization can be used to promote healing and physical well-being by imagining the body healthy and in balance.

Applying the mind-body connection in practice:
- **Cultivate positive thoughts:** Practice gratitude, optimism, and self-compassion, replacing negative thoughts with positive and empowering affirmations.
- **Manage your emotions:** Learn to deal with challenging emotions in a healthy way, using relaxation techniques, mindful breathing, and meditation.
- **Reduce stress:** Identify the factors that cause you stress and develop strategies to deal with them effectively.
- **Practice self-care:** Prioritize your physical and mental health by adopting healthy habits and dedicating time to your well-being.
- **Use visualization:** Imagine your body healthy, strong, and in balance, visualizing healing and physical well-being.

The benefits of harmonizing the mind-body connection:
- **Improved physical health:** Strengthens the immune system, prevents disease, and promotes healing.
- **Emotional well-being:** Increases happiness, self-esteem, and the ability to cope with challenges.
- **Balance and harmony:** Promotes balance between body, mind, and spirit.
- **Increased vital energy:** Increases vitality, disposition, and vital energy.

- **Personal fulfillment:** Leads you to a more fulfilling, authentic, and meaningful life.

Exercise:

Reflect on how your thoughts and emotions influence your physical health. Identify thought and behavior patterns that may be contributing to the imbalance in your mind-body connection. Adopt practices of self-awareness, stress management, and self-care to promote harmony between mind and body.

The mind-body connection is a powerful link that influences your health and well-being. By cultivating positive thoughts, managing your emotions, and taking care of your physical and mental health, you strengthen this connection, promoting healing, balance, and personal fulfillment.

Chapter 33
Deciphering the Body's Signals

In the previous chapter, we explored the profound connection between mind and body. Now, let's delve into the role of emotions in physical health, learning to decipher the signals our body sends us and using this knowledge to promote integral well-being.

Imagine emotions as messengers that bring important information about your internal state. Joy, sadness, anger, fear, love - each emotion carries a message, a signal that the body sends to communicate about your needs, your limits, and your balance.

When we ignore or repress these messages, the body can manifest imbalance through physical symptoms, such as pain, illness, and other health problems. Learning to listen to and interpret these signals is essential to taking care of health in an integral way and promoting well-being at all levels.

Emotions influence physical health in several ways. Chronic stress, for example, can weaken the immune system, increase the risk of heart disease, trigger chronic pain, and affect the functioning of various organs. Repressed anger can manifest as digestive problems, while sadness can lead to fatigue and discouragement.

On the other hand, positive emotions, such as joy, gratitude, and love, strengthen the immune system, promote cardiovascular health, accelerate the healing process, and increase feelings of well-being.

Deciphering the body's signals:
- **Pay attention to physical symptoms:** Headaches, muscle tension, digestive problems, insomnia, changes in appetite - these are just a few examples of how emotions can manifest in the body. Be aware of the signals your body sends you.
- **Identify related emotions:** Try to identify the emotions that may be related to the physical symptoms you are experiencing. Ask yourself: "What am I feeling? What emotions do I have difficulty expressing?"
- **Express your emotions:** Find healthy ways to express your emotions, such as talking to a friend, writing in a journal, practicing artistic activities, or seeking professional help.
- **Manage stress:** Learn to deal with stress effectively using relaxation techniques, mindful breathing, meditation, and physical exercise.
- **Cultivate positive emotions:** Practice gratitude, optimism, compassion, and love, creating a positive inner environment and strengthening your physical and emotional health.
- **Seek professional help:** If you are experiencing persistent or worrisome physical symptoms, see a doctor or other healthcare professional to

investigate the causes and receive appropriate treatment.

The role of emotions in different body systems:

- **Immune system:** Negative emotions can weaken the immune system, making the body more susceptible to disease. Positive emotions strengthen the immune system and increase resistance to disease.
- **Cardiovascular system:** Stress, anger, and anxiety can increase blood pressure and the risk of heart disease. Positive emotions, such as joy and love, promote cardiovascular health.
- **Digestive system:** Anxiety, fear, and anger can affect the digestive system, causing problems such as gastritis, irritable bowel syndrome, and other digestive disorders.
- **Respiratory system:** Anxiety and fear can trigger asthma attacks and other respiratory problems. Relaxation and mindful breathing techniques can help control these symptoms.

Exercise:

Pay attention to the signals your body sends you. Observe your physical symptoms and try to identify the emotions that may be related to them. Adopt practices of self-awareness, stress management, and emotional expression to promote health and integral well-being.

Your body is a complex and interconnected system where emotions play a fundamental role in physical health. By learning to decipher your body's signals and manage your emotions in a healthy way, you become an active agent in promoting your health and integral well-being.

Chapter 34
Self-Regression for Pain Relief

In previous chapters, we uncovered the influence of emotions on physical health. Now, let's explore how self-regression can be a powerful tool for pain relief, allowing you to master pain through the mind and regain control over your body and well-being.

Imagine pain as a warning sign, a request for attention from your body. Self-regression invites you to listen to this message, understand its origin, and use the power of the mind to modulate the perception of pain and promote healing.

Pain is a complex experience that involves both physical and emotional aspects. While the physical sensation of pain is processed by the nervous system, the perception of pain is influenced by factors such as emotions, thoughts, beliefs, and past experiences.

Self-regression empowers you to influence this perception of pain, using techniques to reduce stress, calm the mind, release emotions, and reprogram limiting beliefs that may be amplifying the pain.

Self-regression techniques for pain relief:
- **Mindful breathing:** Deep, slow breathing activates the parasympathetic nervous system,

promoting relaxation, reducing anxiety, and decreasing pain perception.
- **Meditation:** The practice of meditation calms the mind, reduces stress, and promotes the release of endorphins, natural substances that act as pain relievers.
- **Creative visualization:** Imagine the pain dissipating, visualizing your body healthy and in balance. Use positive mental images to promote healing and well-being.
- **Positive affirmations:** Repeat affirmations that reinforce healing and pain relief, such as "My body is healing", "I feel better and better" and "The pain is decreasing".
- **Progressive muscle relaxation:** Tensing and relaxing different muscle groups promotes physical and mental relaxation, reducing tension and pain.
- **Hypnosis:** Hypnosis can be used to access the subconscious and reprogram beliefs and thought patterns that may be contributing to pain.
- **Mindfulness:** The practice of mindfulness invites you to observe pain without judgment, accepting it as part of the present experience and cultivating compassion for yourself.

Applying self-regression for different types of pain:
- **Chronic pain:** Self-regression can help manage chronic pain, reducing pain intensity, improving quality of life, and decreasing dependence on medication.

- **Acute pain:** In cases of acute pain, self-regression can help control pain, promote relaxation, and accelerate the healing process.
- **Emotional pain:** Self-regression can help heal emotional trauma that may be manifesting as physical pain.

Benefits of self-regression for pain relief:
- **Reduction in pain intensity:** Self-regression can help decrease pain intensity, making it more tolerable and less disabling.
- **Improved quality of life:** By reducing pain and suffering, self-regression promotes quality of life and well-being.
- **Reduction of stress and anxiety:** Self-regression techniques promote relaxation, reduce stress and anxiety, which can aggravate pain.
- **Increased self-efficacy:** Self-regression empowers you to take control of your pain and your well-being, increasing your self-efficacy and your confidence in yourself.
- **Reduced dependence on medication:** In some cases, self-regression can help reduce the need for pain medication, or reduce the dosage of medication.

Exercise:

Try self-regression techniques for pain relief. Practice mindful breathing, meditation, visualization, and positive affirmations. Notice how these techniques influence your perception of pain and your well-being.

Self-regression is a powerful ally in pain relief, inviting you to use the power of the mind to modulate pain perception, promote healing, and regain control over your body and well-being.

Chapter 35
Self-Regression Techniques for Chronic Diseases

In the previous chapter, we learned how self-regression can be an ally in pain relief. Now, let's explore how these techniques can be applied to the management of chronic diseases, empowering you to activate your inner healing and live with more quality of life.

Imagine the body as a garden that needs constant care to flourish. Chronic diseases, such as diabetes, hypertension, arthritis and autoimmune diseases, are like challenges that this garden faces, demanding attention, nutrition and specific care.

Self-regression offers tools to strengthen this garden, cultivating resilience, emotional well-being and the mind-body connection, which are pillars for the management of chronic diseases. Through these techniques, you become an active agent in your healing process, complementing conventional medical treatments and promoting a healthier and more balanced life.

It is important to remember that self-regression does not replace traditional medical treatment. It acts as a complement, empowering you to take an active role in your healing process and to deal with the challenges of the disease in a more positive and proactive way.

Self-regression techniques for chronic diseases:

- **Stress management:** Chronic stress can aggravate the symptoms of chronic diseases. Relaxation techniques, such as meditation, mindful breathing and yoga, help control stress and promote well-being.
- **Creative visualization:** Imagine your body healing, visualizing your organs functioning in harmony and your immune system strong and balanced.
- **Positive affirmations:** Repeat affirmations that reinforce healing and well-being, such as "My body is healing every day", "I have strength and vitality" and "I am at peace and harmony".
- **Mindfulness:** The practice of mindfulness invites you to be present in the present moment, accepting your emotions and sensations without judgment and cultivating compassion for yourself.
- **Assertive communication:** Communicate your needs and limits clearly and respectfully, both to healthcare professionals and to your family and friends.
- **Cultivating positive emotions:** Practice gratitude, optimism and love, creating a positive inner environment that strengthens health and well-being.
- **Self-knowledge:** Understand your thought and behavior patterns, identifying how they may be influencing your health and well-being.

- **Healthy habits:** Adopt healthy lifestyle habits, such as a balanced diet, regular physical exercise and restful sleep, which contribute to disease control and overall well-being.

Applying self-regression to different chronic diseases:
- **Diabetes:** Self-regression can help with stress management, emotional regulation and the adoption of healthy habits, which are fundamental for diabetes management.
- **Hypertension:** Relaxation and stress management techniques can contribute to blood pressure control.
- **Autoimmune diseases:** Self-regression can help strengthen the immune system, reduce inflammation and promote emotional well-being.
- **Heart disease:** Stress management, healthy eating and exercise, combined with self-regression techniques, can help prevent and treat heart disease.
- **Cancer:** Self-regression can complement cancer treatment, helping to cope with stress, anxiety and the side effects of treatment, in addition to promoting quality of life and emotional well-being.

Benefits of self-regression for chronic diseases:
- **Improved quality of life:** Promotes physical, emotional and social well-being, improving quality of life and the ability to cope with illness.

- **Reduced stress and anxiety:** Helps control stress, anxiety and depression, which can aggravate the symptoms of chronic diseases.
- **Strengthening the immune system:** Stimulates the immune system, increasing resistance to disease and infection.
- **Increased self-efficacy:** Empowers you to take an active role in your healing process, increasing your self-confidence and your ability to deal with the challenges of the disease.
- **Complementation of medical treatment:** Self-regression acts as a complement to conventional medical treatments, promoting healing and integral well-being.

Exercise:

If you live with a chronic illness, try self-regression techniques to strengthen your health and well-being. Practice stress management, creative visualization, positive affirmations and mindfulness. Adopt healthy lifestyle habits and cultivate positive emotions.

Self-regression is a powerful ally in the management of chronic diseases, inviting you to activate your inner healing, strengthen your resilience and live with more quality of life, even in the face of the challenges of the disease.

Chapter 36
Self-Regression and the Immune System

In previous chapters, we explored the power of self-regression to deal with pain and chronic diseases. Now, let's turn our attention to the immune system, discovering how self-regression can strengthen the body's defenses and promote health in an integral way.

Imagine the immune system as an army of guardians that protect your body against invaders, such as viruses, bacteria and other pathogens. Self-regression acts as a commander who trains and strengthens this army, equipping it with the best weapons to fight disease and keep the body healthy and balanced.

The immune system is a complex network of cells, tissues and organs that work together to defend the body against disease. [1] It is responsible for identifying and destroying invading agents, repairing damaged tissues and maintaining the body's balance.

Self-regression, through its various techniques, can positively influence the immune system, reducing stress, balancing emotions, promoting relaxation and cultivating positivity, factors that contribute to strengthening the body's defenses.

How self-regression strengthens the immune system:
- **Stress reduction:** Chronic stress is one of the main enemies of the immune system, weakening its defenses and making the body more susceptible to disease. Relaxation techniques, such as meditation, mindful breathing and yoga, help control stress and strengthen the immune system.
- **Emotional balance:** Negative emotions, such as fear, anger and sadness, can negatively affect the immune system. Self-regression, through emotional management, promotes emotional balance and strengthens the body's defenses.
- **Improved sleep quality:** Restful sleep is essential for the proper functioning of the immune system. Self-regression, through relaxation and visualization techniques, can help improve sleep quality.
- **Cultivating positive thoughts:** Positive thoughts and empowering beliefs strengthen the immune system, while negative thoughts and limiting beliefs can weaken it. Self-regression, through positive affirmations and creative visualization, cultivates positivity and strengthens the body's defenses.
- **Healthy habits:** Self-regression can help you adopt healthy lifestyle habits, such as a balanced diet, regular physical exercise and contact with nature, which contribute to strengthening the immune system.

Self-regression techniques to strengthen the immune system:
- **Meditation:** The practice of meditation reduces stress, promotes relaxation and increases the production of the body's defense cells.
- **Mindful breathing:** Deep, slow breathing calms the nervous system, reduces anxiety and strengthens the immune system.
- **Creative visualization:** Imagine your immune system strong and efficient, fighting disease and keeping your body healthy.
- **Positive affirmations:** Repeat affirmations that reinforce the health and strength of your immune system, such as "My immune system is strong and powerful", "My body is protected" and "I am healthy and vibrant".
- **Yoga and Tai Chi Chuan:** These practices combine gentle movements, mindful breathing and meditation, promoting physical, mental and emotional balance, and strengthening the immune system.
- **Contact with nature:** Spending time in contact with nature, such as walking in parks, gardens or forests, reduces stress, increases the feeling of well-being and strengthens the immune system.

Benefits of self-regression for the immune system:
- **Increased resistance to disease:** Strengthens the body's defenses, making it more resistant to viruses, bacteria and other pathogens.

- **Disease prevention:** Helps prevent disease by reducing the risk of infections and other health problems.
- **Improved overall health:** Promotes physical, mental and emotional health, contributing to overall well-being.
- **Acceleration of the healing process:** In case of illness, self-regression can help accelerate the healing process, strengthening the immune system and promoting recovery.
- **Increased vitality:** Increases vital energy, disposition and the feeling of well-being.

Exercise:

Incorporate self-regression techniques into your daily routine to strengthen your immune system. Practice meditation, mindful breathing, visualization and positive affirmations. Adopt healthy lifestyle habits and cultivate positive emotions.

Self-regression is a powerful ally in the pursuit of a healthier and more balanced life. By strengthening your immune system through these techniques, you increase your resistance to disease, promote healing and cultivate overall well-being.

Chapter 37
Conscious and Intuitive Eating

In previous chapters, we strengthened the immune system through self-regression. Now, let's turn our attention to food, discovering how the practice of conscious and intuitive eating can nourish not only the body, but also the soul, promoting health, well-being and a more harmonious relationship with food.

Imagine eating as an act of love and respect for yourself, a moment of connection with your body and with nature. Conscious and intuitive eating invites you to abandon restrictive diets and guilt, and to reconnect with your body's hunger and satiety signals, choosing foods that nourish you and give you pleasure.

Mindful eating involves paying full attention to the act of eating, savoring each food, chewing carefully and appreciating the flavors, aromas and textures. It is an invitation to slow down, to connect with the present moment and to honor the wisdom of your body.

Intuitive eating, in turn, encourages you to trust your internal hunger and satiety signals, eating when you are hungry and stopping when you are satisfied, without rules or restrictions. It is a process of reconnecting with your intuition, learning to distinguish physical hunger from emotional hunger and making food choices that nourish you on all levels.

Principles of Conscious and Intuitive Eating:

- **Reject the diet mentality:** Abandon restrictive diets and the incessant pursuit of the perfect body. Focus on nourishing your body with healthy foods and cultivating a positive relationship with food.
- **Honor your hunger:** Pay attention to your body's hunger signals and eat when you are hungry, without depriving yourself or blaming yourself.
- **Make peace with food:** Allow yourself to eat all the foods you like, without restrictions or judgments. Trust your ability to make conscious and balanced choices.
- **Challenge the "food police":** Silence the inner critical voice that judges you for your food choices. Cultivate self-compassion and freedom of choice.
- **Feel satiety:** Pay attention to your body's satiety signals and stop eating when you are satisfied, even if there is still food on your plate.
- **Discover the satisfaction factor:** Choose foods that give you pleasure and satisfaction, in addition to nourishing your body.
- **Deal with emotions without using food:** Find healthy ways to deal with your emotions, without resorting to food as a form of escape or comfort.
- **Respect your body:** Accept and love your body as it is, regardless of its size or shape.

- **Exercise to feel good:** Practice physical activities that give you pleasure and well-being, without focusing only on weight loss or aesthetics.
- **Honor your health:** Make food choices that contribute to your health and well-being in the long term, without radicalism or extremism.

Benefits of Conscious and Intuitive Eating:
- **Improved relationship with food:** Promotes a healthier and more balanced relationship with food, free from guilt, restrictions and compulsions.
- **Physical health:** Contributes to physical health by providing the necessary nutrients for the proper functioning of the body.
- **Emotional well-being:** Reduces anxiety, stress and depression, promoting emotional well-being and self-acceptance.
- **Self-knowledge:** Increases body awareness, connection with intuition and the ability to recognize and honor your body's needs.
- **Balance and harmony:** Promotes balance between body, mind and soul, cultivating a more harmonious and fulfilling life.

Exercise:

Start practicing conscious and intuitive eating today. Pay attention to your body's hunger and satiety signals, savor each food with full attention and make food choices that nourish you and give you pleasure.

Conscious and intuitive eating is a path of self-knowledge, healing and liberation. By reconnecting with your body's wisdom and honoring its needs, you cultivate a more harmonious relationship with food and nourish body and soul in perfect harmony.

Chapter 38
Conscious Movement

In previous chapters, we learned to nourish body and soul through mindful eating. Now, let's get the body moving and explore the benefits of exercise for health, well-being and self-regression.

Imagine the body as a musical instrument that needs to be tuned and played to express its unique melody. Physical exercise is like musical practice, which tunes the body, releases tension, increases vital energy and puts you in tune with the rhythm of life.

Physical exercise goes beyond the pursuit of aesthetics or athletic performance. It is an act of self-care, a way to honor your body, to celebrate your vitality and to connect with your inner strength.

Whatever your favorite activity - walking, dancing, swimming, running, practicing yoga or weight training - the important thing is to find the movement that makes you feel good, that energizes you and puts you in touch with the joy of moving.

Conscious movement for a healthier life:
- **Find an activity you enjoy:** Try different types of physical exercise and discover which one gives you the most pleasure and satisfaction.

- **Move with full attention:** Pay attention to your body during practice, observing your sensations, your limits and your natural rhythm.
- **Connect with nature:** Take the opportunity to exercise outdoors, in contact with nature, absorbing the energy of the sun, fresh air and the beauty of the environment.
- **Listen to your body:** Respect your limits and don't push yourself beyond what your body can handle. Adjust the intensity and duration of your workouts according to your needs and physical condition.
- **Vary your workouts:** Try different types of exercise to work different muscle groups and avoid monotony.
- **Find a workout partner:** Exercising with a friend or family member can increase motivation and enjoyment of the practice.
- **Incorporate movement into your daily life:** Use the stairs instead of the elevator, walk or bike instead of using the car, take short breaks to stretch during work.
- **Celebrate your progress:** Recognize and celebrate every achievement, no matter how small. The celebration motivates you to keep moving and to seek a healthier life.

Benefits of exercise for self-regression:

- **Reduced stress and anxiety:** Exercise releases endorphins, substances that promote well-being and reduce stress and anxiety.

- **Improved mood:** Regular physical exercise helps fight depression and promote good mood.
- **Increased self-esteem:** Physical exercise contributes to improving self-esteem and self-confidence, by promoting health, vitality and a sense of well-being.
- **Improved concentration and focus:** The practice of physical exercise improves concentration, focus and memory, contributing to cognitive performance.
- **Increased vital energy:** Physical exercise increases vital energy, disposition and vitality.
- **Improved sleep quality:** Regular physical exercise contributes to improving sleep quality, promoting relaxation and restful sleep.
- **Mind-body connection:** Physical exercise promotes the mind-body connection, increasing body awareness and perception of body signals.

Exercise:

Incorporate conscious movement into your life. Find an activity you enjoy and practice it regularly, paying attention to your body and celebrating your progress.

Movement is life. By moving consciously, you nourish your body, calm your mind and connect with your inner strength, cultivating a healthier, more balanced and happier life.

Chapter 39
Techniques for Better Sleep

In the previous chapters, we put the body in motion and explored the benefits of physical exercise. Now, let's prepare for a well-deserved rest and discover how to cultivate restful sleep, essential for health, well-being, and self-regression.

Imagine sleep as a deep dive into an ocean of tranquility, where the body and mind regenerate, energies are renewed, and the soul reconnects with its essence. Sleeping well is like recharging your batteries, allowing you to wake up refreshed, energized, and ready to live each day with more vitality and willingness.

Sleep is an essential physiological state for life, as important as food and exercise. During sleep, the body and mind recover from the wear and tear of everyday life, consolidate memories, regulate hormones, and restore energy.

Sleep quality directly impacts your physical and mental health, influencing your mood, concentration, creativity, immune system, and ability to cope with stress.

Cultivating restful sleep is like creating a sanctuary of peace and tranquility, where you can surrender to rest and awaken renewed for a fuller and more balanced life.

Techniques for better sleep:

- **Create a relaxing bedtime routine:** Establish a relaxing ritual before bed, such as taking a warm bath, reading a book, listening to calm music, or practicing meditation.
- **Prepare your sleep environment:** Ensure your bedroom is conducive to sleep, with a comfortable temperature, low light, and silence. Invest in a comfortable mattress and pillows.
- **Disconnect from electronics:** Avoid using electronics such as cell phones, tablets, and computers for at least an hour before bed. The blue light emitted by these devices can interfere with the production of melatonin, [1] the sleep hormone.
- **Eat lightly at night:** Avoid heavy and stimulating meals before bed. Opt for light and easily digestible foods.
- **Exercise regularly:** Regular physical activity contributes to better sleep quality, but avoid exercising too close to bedtime.
- **Manage stress:** Stress and anxiety are enemies of sleep. Practice relaxation techniques, such as meditation, mindful breathing, and yoga, to calm the mind and body before bed.
- **Avoid caffeine and alcohol:** Caffeine and alcohol can interfere with sleep quality. Avoid consuming these substances at night.

- **Get sunlight during the day:** Sunlight helps regulate the circadian cycle, which controls the rhythm of sleep. Get some sunlight during the day, especially in the morning.
- **Keep a sleep diary:** Record your sleep habits, bedtimes and wake-up times, and the quality of your sleep. This can help you identify patterns and make adjustments to your routine to sleep better.
- **Consult a specialist:** If you suffer from insomnia or other sleep disorders, seek a doctor or sleep specialist for proper guidance and treatment.

Benefits of restful sleep for self-regression:
- **Improved physical and mental health:** Restful sleep contributes to physical and mental health, strengthening the immune system, regulating mood, increasing concentration and memory, and promoting overall well-being.
- **Increased vital energy:** Sleeping well gives you more energy, willingness, and vitality to live each day more intensely.
- **Improved ability to cope with stress:** Restful sleep increases your ability to cope with stress, anxiety, and life's challenges.
- **Increased creativity and intuition:** During sleep, the subconscious processes information and connects you with your intuition and creativity.
- **Improved mind-body connection:** Restful sleep promotes harmony between mind and body, allowing you to connect with your inner signals and promote self-knowledge.

Exercise:

Assess the quality of your sleep and adopt techniques to sleep better. Create a relaxing bedtime routine, prepare your sleep environment, and practice relaxation techniques to calm your mind and body.

Restful sleep is a gift you give yourself, a moment of deep connection with your body and soul. By cultivating healthy sleep habits, you nurture your health, renew your energies, and awaken to a fuller and more balanced life.

Chapter 40
Detoxification of Body and Mind

In the previous chapters, we learned the importance of restful sleep for health and well-being. Now, let's deepen the self-care journey and explore the detoxification of the body and mind, an essential process to purify energies, renew cells, and promote integral balance.

Imagine the body as a river that, over time, accumulates impurities and toxins from pollution, inadequate diet, stress, and other factors. Detoxification is like a deep cleaning of this river, removing waste, purifying the waters, and allowing vital energy to flow freely.

Body detoxification involves eliminating accumulated toxins through healthy habits such as natural eating, drinking pure water, exercising, and using purification techniques such as detox juices and diuretic teas.

Mind detoxification, in turn, focuses on releasing negative thoughts, limiting beliefs, and toxic emotions that may be blocking your energy flow and hindering your personal growth.

Purifying the body:

- **Natural food:** Prioritize organic foods, fruits, vegetables, and whole grains, rich in nutrients and antioxidants that help eliminate toxins.
- **Hydration:** Drink plenty of pure water to help eliminate toxins through urine and sweat.
- **Physical exercise:** Regular physical exercise stimulates blood circulation, the elimination of toxins through sweat, and the oxygenation of cells.
- **Detox juices:** Include detox juices based on fruits, vegetables, and greens in your diet to help eliminate toxins and revitalize the body.
- **Diuretic teas:** Consume diuretic teas, such as green tea, hibiscus, and horsetail, to help eliminate fluids and toxins through urine.
- **Detox baths:** Take baths with Epsom salts or clay to help eliminate toxins through the skin.
- **Sauna:** The sauna helps eliminate toxins through sweat and promotes muscle relaxation.

Purifying the mind:
- **Meditation:** The practice of meditation calms the mind, reduces stress, and promotes the release of negative thoughts and emotions.
- **Mindfulness:** Cultivate mindfulness in your daily life, observing your thoughts and emotions without judgment and connecting with the present moment.
- **Positive affirmations:** Repeat affirmations that promote the release of negative thoughts and the purification of the mind, such as "I release all

thoughts and emotions that no longer serve me" and "My mind is at peace and harmony."
- **Forgiveness:** Practice forgiveness, releasing grudges, resentments, and guilt that may be overburdening you.
- **Contact with nature:** Spend time in contact with nature, breathing fresh air, contemplating the beauty of the environment, and connecting with the vital energy of the earth.
- **Creative expression:** Express your emotions through art, music, writing, or other forms of creative expression, releasing blocked energies and promoting the purification of the mind.

Benefits of body and mind detoxification:
- **Increased vital energy:** Detoxification promotes the renewal of energies, increasing vitality, willingness, and well-being.
- **Improved physical health:** Eliminates toxins from the body, strengthens the immune system, improves digestion, and promotes physical health.
- **Emotional balance:** Releases negative emotions, reduces stress and anxiety, and promotes emotional balance.
- **Mental clarity:** Increases mental clarity, focus, and concentration.
- **Self-knowledge:** Promotes self-knowledge, connection with intuition, and the ability to self-regulate.
- **Integral well-being:** Contributes to integral well-being, harmonizing body, mind, and spirit.

Exercise:

Incorporate body and mind detoxification habits into your routine. Adopt a natural diet, hydrate, exercise, cultivate mindfulness and positivity, and express your emotions in a healthy way.

The detoxification of body and mind is a continuous process of purification and renewal, which invites you to take care of yourself on all levels and cultivate a lighter, healthier, and more balanced life.

Chapter 41
Hormonal Balance and Self-Regression

In the previous chapters, we purified the body and mind through detoxification. Now, let's delve into the endocrine system and discover how self-regression can help with hormonal balance, promoting inner harmony and a fuller life.

Imagine hormones as chemical messengers that travel through the body, regulating various essential functions, such as growth, metabolism, mood, sleep, and reproduction. Hormonal balance is like a tuned orchestra, where each hormone plays its role in harmony with the others, ensuring the proper functioning of the body.

Self-regression, through its various techniques, can help with hormonal regulation by reducing stress, balancing emotions, promoting relaxation, and cultivating healthy habits - factors that directly influence the endocrine system.

Hormonal imbalances can cause several physical and emotional symptoms, such as mood swings, anxiety, depression, fatigue, insomnia, weight gain, skin problems, and menstrual irregularities. Self-regression can be an ally in managing these symptoms, complementing conventional medical treatments and promoting overall well-being.

How self-regression contributes to hormonal balance:
- **Stress management:** Chronic stress is one of the main factors contributing to hormonal imbalance. Relaxation techniques such as meditation, mindful breathing, and yoga help control stress and promote hormonal harmony.
- **Emotional balance:** Emotions such as anxiety, fear, and anger can affect hormone production. Self-regression, through emotional management, promotes emotional balance and contributes to hormonal regulation.
- **Improved sleep quality:** Restful sleep is essential for proper hormone production. Self-regression, through relaxation and visualization techniques, can help improve sleep quality.
- **Healthy eating:** A balanced diet, rich in nutrients and vitamins, is essential for the proper functioning of the endocrine system. Self-regression, through mindful eating, can help you adopt healthy eating habits.
- **Physical exercise:** Regular physical exercise contributes to hormonal balance, in addition to promoting physical and mental health.
- **Mind-body connection:** Self-regression promotes the mind-body connection, increasing body awareness and perception of body signals, which can help identify hormonal imbalances.

Self-regression techniques for hormonal balance:
- **Meditation:** The practice of meditation reduces stress, promotes relaxation, and balances the nervous system, contributing to hormonal regulation.
- **Mindful breathing:** Deep, slow breathing calms the nervous system, reduces anxiety, and promotes hormonal balance.
- **Creative visualization:** Imagine your hormones in balance, visualizing your body functioning in harmony and your endocrine organs healthy.
- **Positive affirmations:** Repeat affirmations that reinforce hormonal balance and the health of your endocrine system, such as "My hormones are in perfect balance", "My body is healthy and in harmony" and "I feel balanced and at peace".
- **Yoga and Tai Chi Chuan:** These practices combine gentle movements, mindful breathing, and meditation, promoting physical, mental, and emotional balance, and contributing to hormonal regulation.
- **Aromatherapy:** The use of essential oils, such as lavender, chamomile, and geranium, can help with hormonal balance and relieve symptoms related to hormonal imbalances.

Benefits of self-regression for hormonal balance:
- **Symptom relief:** Helps relieve symptoms related to hormonal imbalances, such as mood swings, anxiety, depression, fatigue, and insomnia.

- **Improved physical health:** Promotes physical health by regulating metabolism, sleep, digestion, and other important bodily functions.
- **Emotional balance:** Contributes to emotional balance, reducing stress, anxiety, and promoting mental well-being.
- **Increased vitality:** Increases vital energy, disposition, and vitality.
- **Improved quality of life:** Promotes quality of life by increasing physical, emotional, and social well-being.

Exercise:

Incorporate self-regression techniques into your daily routine to promote hormonal balance. Practice meditation, mindful breathing, visualization, and positive affirmations. Adopt healthy lifestyle habits, such as a balanced diet, regular exercise, and restful sleep.

Self-regression is a powerful ally in the search for hormonal balance and inner harmony. By cultivating self-knowledge, stress management, and healthy habits, you contribute to hormonal regulation and promote a fuller and more balanced life.

Chapter 42
Self-Regression for Mental Health

In the previous chapters, we sought inner harmony through hormonal balance. Now, let's turn our attention to mental health and discover how self-regression can be a powerful ally in cultivating inner balance, peace of mind, and emotional well-being.

Imagine the mind as a garden that needs to be cared for with attention and affection to flourish. Mental health is like the fertility of this garden, allowing positive thoughts, balanced emotions, and healthy relationships to flourish in their fullness.

Self-regression offers tools to cultivate this inner garden, removing the weeds of negative thoughts, cultivating the flowers of positivity, and nourishing the soil of your mind with self-knowledge, resilience, and compassion.

In an increasingly fast-paced and challenging world, taking care of mental health is essential to deal with stress, anxiety, depression, and other emotional challenges. Self-regression empowers you to take control of your mind, cultivate inner balance, and build a happier and more meaningful life.

How self-regression contributes to mental health:

- **Stress management:** Chronic stress is one of the main factors contributing to the development of mental health problems. Relaxation techniques, such as meditation, mindful breathing, and yoga, help control stress and promote emotional well-being.
- **Emotional regulation:** Self-regression helps you identify, understand, and manage your emotions in a healthy way, preventing negative emotions from dominating you and affecting your mental health.
- **Self-knowledge:** Through self-observation and introspection, self-regression leads you to a deep self-knowledge, allowing you to understand your thought patterns, your beliefs and your behaviors, and promoting self-acceptance and self-love.
- **Empowering beliefs:** Self-regression helps you identify and transform limiting beliefs that may be sabotaging your mental health and well-being. Through positive affirmations and creative visualization, you cultivate empowering beliefs that propel you toward a happier and more fulfilling life.
- **Resilience:** Self-regression strengthens your resilience, increasing your ability to deal with adversity, overcome challenges, and adapt to change with more flexibility and optimism.
- **Healthy relationships:** Self-regression helps you build healthier relationships based on assertive communication, empathy, and mutual respect.

Self-regression techniques for mental health:

- **Meditation:** The practice of meditation calms the mind, reduces anxiety, increases concentration, and promotes inner peace.
- **Mindfulness:** Mindfulness invites you to be present in the present moment, observing your thoughts and emotions without judgment, cultivating acceptance and compassion for yourself.
- **Mindful breathing:** Deep, slow breathing calms the nervous system, reduces stress, and promotes relaxation.
- **Yoga:** The practice of yoga combines physical postures, breathing exercises, and meditation, promoting physical, mental, and emotional balance.
- **Therapeutic writing:** Writing about your thoughts and emotions in a journal can help you process feelings, organize ideas, and promote self-understanding.
- **Positive affirmations:** Repeat affirmations that promote mental health, emotional well-being, and self-confidence, such as "I am strong", "I am capable" and "I deserve to be happy".
- **Creative visualization:** Imagine yourself at peace, balanced and happy, visualizing the realization of your dreams and overcoming your challenges.

Benefits of self-regression for mental health:
- **Reduction of stress and anxiety:** Promotes relaxation, reduces anxiety and stress, and

increases the ability to deal with challenging situations.
- **Mood improvement:** Helps fight depression, increase self-esteem and promote good humor.
- **Increased self-awareness:** Promotes self-knowledge, self-acceptance and self-love.
- **Strengthening resilience:** Increases the ability to deal with adversity and overcome challenges.
- **Improvement in relationships:** Contributes to building healthier and more authentic relationships.
- **Prevention of mental illness:** Helps prevent the development of mental disorders, such as anxiety and depression.

Exercise:

Incorporate self-regression techniques into your daily routine to cultivate inner balance and promote mental health. Practice meditation, mindfulness, mindful breathing, and positive affirmations. Cultivate self-knowledge, resilience, and healthy relationships.

Self-regression is a powerful ally in the pursuit of mental health and emotional well-being. By cultivating inner balance, you become stronger, more resilient and happier, able to deal with life's challenges with serenity and wisdom.

Chapter 43
Prevention and Health Promotion

In the previous chapters, we addressed various aspects of physical and mental health. Now, let's integrate this knowledge and explore how self-regression can be a path to disease prevention and health promotion, cultivating overall well-being and a healthier and more balanced life.

Imagine health as a state of complete physical, mental and social well-being, and not just the absence of disease. Self-regression invites you to take an active role in building your health, adopting healthy habits, cultivating self-knowledge and using the power of the mind to promote balance and harmony at all levels of your being.

Disease prevention focuses on preventing the onset of health problems through the adoption of healthy habits, vaccination, preventive exams and other care. Health promotion, in turn, goes beyond prevention, seeking to create conditions for people to reach their maximum potential for health and well-being.

Self-regression, with its tools for self-knowledge, stress management, emotional regulation and cultivation of positivity, becomes a powerful ally in the prevention and promotion of health, empowering you to build a healthier, more balanced and happy life.

Self-regression as a path to integral health:
- **Self-knowledge:** Understand your thought patterns, your emotions, your behaviors and your needs, so that you can make more conscious choices aligned with your health and well-being.
- **Stress management:** Chronic stress is one of the main risk factors for various diseases. Use relaxation techniques, such as meditation, mindful breathing and yoga, to control stress and promote physical and mental health.
- **Emotional regulation:** Negative emotions, such as anxiety, fear and anger, can negatively affect health. Self-regression helps you deal with your emotions in a healthy way, cultivating emotional balance and well-being.
- **Healthy habits:** Self-regression helps you adopt healthy lifestyle habits, such as a balanced diet, regular exercise, restful sleep and contact with nature.
- **Positive thoughts:** Cultivate positive thoughts, empowering beliefs and optimistic attitudes, which contribute to mental health, emotional well-being and disease prevention.
- **Resilience:** Strengthen your resilience, increasing your ability to deal with adversity, overcome challenges and adapt to change with more flexibility and positivity.
- **Healthy relationships:** Cultivate healthy relationships based on assertive communication,

empathy and mutual respect, which contribute to emotional and social well-being.
- **Disease prevention:** Use self-regression to strengthen your immune system, prevent disease and promote physical and mental health.

Applying self-regression in the prevention and promotion of health:
- **Mindful eating:** Practice mindful eating, paying attention to your body's hunger and satiety cues, choosing nutritious foods and cultivating a healthy relationship with food.
- **Physical exercise:** Incorporate physical exercise into your routine, choosing activities that give you pleasure and that are in accordance with your physical conditions.
- **Restful sleep:** Cultivate healthy sleep habits by creating a relaxing bedtime routine and ensuring an environment conducive to rest.
- **Time management:** Organize your time efficiently, prioritizing your activities and avoiding overload, which can lead to stress and imbalance.
- **Connection with nature:** Spend time in contact with nature, breathing fresh air, contemplating the beauty of the environment and connecting with the vital energy of the earth.
- **Integrative practices:** Experiment with integrative practices, such as yoga, meditation, acupuncture and massage, which can complement health care and promote overall well-being.

Benefits of self-regression for the prevention and promotion of health:
- **Increased quality of life:** Promotes a healthier, more balanced and happy life.
- **Disease prevention:** Reduces the risk of developing physical and mental illness.
- **Improved physical and mental health:** Strengthens the immune system, improves mood, increases concentration and promotes general well-being.
- **Increased self-efficacy:** Empowers you to take control of your health and well-being.
- **Personal development:** Promotes self-knowledge, personal growth and the realization of your potentials.

Exercise:

Reflect on your lifestyle habits and identify which areas you can improve to promote your health and well-being. Incorporate self-regression techniques into your daily routine, cultivating self-knowledge, stress management, emotional regulation, and positivity.

Self-regression is a path to integral health, inviting you to be the protagonist of your health and well-being. By cultivating healthy habits, using the power of the mind and connecting with your inner wisdom, you build a fuller, more balanced and happy life.

Chapter 44
Spirituality and Self-Knowledge

In the previous chapters, we built a path to integral well-being through the prevention and promotion of health. Now, let's transcend the limits of the physical body and mind, and explore the spiritual dimension of the human being, discovering how spirituality and self-knowledge intertwine to awaken the essence of being and lead to a deeper and more meaningful life.

Imagine spirituality as a compass that guides you towards your life purpose, connecting you with something greater than yourself, whatever your belief or spiritual path. It is the search for meaning, connection and transcendence, which drives you to explore the depths of your being and connect with your divine essence.

Self-knowledge, in turn, is the lantern that illuminates the path of your spiritual journey, revealing your deepest values, beliefs, emotions and motivations. It is through self-knowledge that you become aware of who you truly are, your potential and your life purpose.

The union between spirituality and self-knowledge is like a sacred dance, where the search for connection with the divine intertwines with the journey of self-discovery, leading to a more authentic, compassionate and meaningful life.

Awakening to the essence of being:
- **Explore your spirituality:** Seek a spiritual path that resonates with your values and beliefs, whether through religion, meditation, contact with nature or other practices that connect you with the sacred.
- **Cultivate connection with the divine:** Take time to connect with your spirituality, whether through prayer, meditation, contemplation of nature, or other practices that inspire and uplift you.
- **Practice introspection:** Set aside moments of stillness and introspection to connect with your inner world, observe your thoughts and emotions, and ask yourself about your values, beliefs, and life purpose.
- **Study and learn:** Seek knowledge about different spiritual traditions, philosophies and practices that will help you on your journey of self-knowledge and spiritual development.
- **Connect with nature:** Spend time in contact with nature, contemplating the beauty of the natural world, breathing fresh air and energizing yourself with the life force of the earth.
- **Practice compassion:** Cultivate compassion for yourself and others, recognizing the interconnectedness of all beings and seeking to act with love, kindness and respect.
- **Live with purpose:** Seek to live a life of purpose, aligned with your values and your soul mission.

Find meaning in your actions and contribute to the good of the world.
- **Trust your intuition:** Learn to listen to the voice of your intuition, which guides you towards your path and connects you with your inner wisdom.

Benefits of spirituality and self-knowledge:
- **Inner peace:** Cultivates inner peace, serenity and harmony in your life.
- **Life purpose:** Helps you find your life purpose and live with more meaning and fulfillment.
- **Resilience:** Strengthens your resilience, increasing your ability to deal with adversity and overcome challenges with faith and hope.
- **Compassion and love:** Awakens compassion, unconditional love and connection with all beings.
- **Self-knowledge:** Promotes self-knowledge, self-acceptance and self-love.
- **Connection with the divine:** Strengthens your connection with the divine, whatever your belief or spiritual path.
- **Integral well-being:** Contributes to integral well-being, harmonizing body, mind and spirit.

Exercise:

Reflect on your spirituality and how it connects with your self-knowledge. Explore different spiritual paths, cultivate connection with the divine, and practice introspection to connect with your essence and live with more purpose and meaning.

Spirituality and self-knowledge are like two wings that lift you towards your true essence, connecting you with the divine and leading you to a fuller, more compassionate and meaningful life.

Chapter 45
Revitalizing Body and Soul

In the previous chapters, we awakened to the essence of being through spirituality and self-knowledge. Now, let's reconnect with the primordial source of energy and vitality: nature. We will explore how connecting with the natural world can revitalize body and soul, promote healing and well-being, and deepen your self-regression journey.

Imagine nature as a big welcoming hug, a refuge of peace and serenity that reconnects you with your essence and nourishes you on all levels. Nature is our original home, the cradle of life, the source of vital energy that sustains and inspires us.

Throughout history, human beings have always been connected to nature, depending on it for their survival and finding inspiration, healing, and spiritual connection in it. However, with the accelerated pace of modern life and increasing urbanization, we often distance ourselves from this vital source, losing touch with our essence and the natural rhythm of life.

Reconnecting with nature is like returning home, rediscovering your roots, and nourishing yourself with the vital energy that emanates from every tree, every river, every mountain, and every creature. It is an invitation to awaken the senses, calm the mind, breathe fresh air, and reconnect with the ancestral wisdom of the earth.

Revitalizing body and soul in nature:
- **Immerse yourself in nature:** Set aside time to be in contact with nature, whether in parks, gardens, forests, beaches, or mountains. Walk barefoot on the grass, hug a tree, contemplate the sunrise or sunset, listen to the birds singing, feel the breeze on your face.
- **Awaken your senses:** Pay attention to the sounds, smells, colors, and textures of nature. Observe the details, the nuances, the beauty, and diversity of the natural world.
- **Breathe deeply:** Breathe in the fresh air of nature, filling your lungs with the vital energy that emanates from plants and trees.
- **Connect with the earth:** Sit or lie down on the ground, feeling the connection with the vital energy of the planet. Imagine your roots connecting with the roots of the trees, absorbing the strength and stability of the earth.
- **Meditate in nature:** Find a quiet place in nature to meditate, connecting with the peace and serenity of the environment.
- **Engage in outdoor activities:** Walk, run, swim, practice yoga, or other physical activities in contact with nature.
- **Grow plants:** Grow plants at home or in the garden, caring for them with affection and

observing the cycle of life manifest in each sprout, flower, and fruit.
- **Connect with animals:** Observe animals in their natural habitat, learning from their wisdom and being inspired by their connection to nature.
- **Give thanks for nature:** Cultivate gratitude for the beauty, abundance, and wisdom of nature. Recognize the interdependence between all living beings and the importance of caring for the planet.

Benefits of connecting with nature for self-regression:

- **Stress reduction:** Contact with nature reduces stress, anxiety, and depression, promoting relaxation and mental well-being.
- **Improved physical health:** Increases immunity, improves sleep quality, reduces blood pressure, and promotes cardiovascular health.
- **Increased creativity:** Stimulates creativity, intuition, and connection with your inner wisdom.
- **Elevated consciousness:** Promotes the expansion of consciousness, connection with the divine, and spiritual awakening.
- **Self-knowledge:** Facilitates self-knowledge, introspection, and connection with your essence.
- **Emotional healing:** Assists in healing traumas, releasing negative emotions, and promoting emotional balance.
- **Energy renewal:** Revitalizes body and soul, increasing vital energy and disposition.

Exercise:

Take some time to connect with nature today. Walk in a park, sit in a garden, contemplate the sky, listen to the birds singing, breathe fresh air, and feel the vital energy of the earth revitalizing you.

Nature is an inexhaustible source of healing, wisdom, and inspiration. By connecting with the natural world, you reconnect with your essence, revitalize body and soul, and deepen your self-regression journey towards a fuller and more balanced life.

Chapter 46
Developing Intuition

In the previous chapters, we reconnected with the source of vital energy through nature. Now, let's turn our attention inward and explore the power of intuition, that inner voice that whispers wisdom and guidance on our path. We will learn to listen to this subtle voice, trust its insights, and use it as a compass on our self-regression journey.

Imagine intuition as an internal radar, an antenna that captures information beyond the five senses, tuning into subtle frequencies and revealing knowledge that transcends logic and reason. It is the voice of your inner self, of your soul, that guides you with wisdom and connects you with your deepest truth.

Intuition manifests itself in different ways: a hunch, a feeling, an image, a sudden idea, a soft voice whispering the direction to follow. Often, it arises in moments of stillness, when we silence the whirlwind of thoughts and open ourselves to inner wisdom.

Developing intuition is like tuning a musical instrument, adjusting the strings of your perception to capture the subtle melodies of your soul. It is learning to trust your instincts, recognize the signs that the universe sends you, and follow your inner voice with confidence and courage.

Opening yourself to the voice of intuition:
- **Quiet the mind:** Intuition manifests itself more clearly when the mind is calm and receptive. Practice meditation, mindfulness, and other relaxation techniques to silence the internal dialogue and connect with your center.
- **Pay attention to your feelings:** Intuition often manifests itself through subtle feelings and sensations. Pay attention to your body, your emotions, and your hunches. What is your heart telling you?
- **Trust your instincts:** When an intuition arises, don't ignore or rationalize it. Trust your instincts and follow your inner voice, even if it doesn't make logical sense at the time.
- **Observe the signs:** The universe communicates with us through signs and synchronicities. Be aware of the events, people, and messages that cross your path, as they may contain important clues and guidance.
- **Cultivate curiosity:** Ask questions to your inner self, seeking answers and insights. Keep an open and curious mind, allowing intuition to guide you in new directions.
- **Write down your intuitions:** Keep a journal to record your intuitions, dreams, and insights. This will help you recognize the patterns of your intuition and strengthen your connection with it.

- **Experiment:** Test your intuitions in small, everyday decisions. The more you trust your intuition, the stronger it will become.
- **Be patient:** Developing intuition is a gradual process that takes time and practice. Be patient with yourself and trust that your intuition will become increasingly clear and accurate.

Benefits of developing intuition:
- **Wiser decision-making:** Intuition helps you make decisions that are more aligned with your values and life purpose.
- **Self-knowledge:** Intuition connects you with your inner wisdom, revealing your deepest desires, needs, and potentials.
- **Creativity:** Intuition opens doors to creativity, inspiration, and innovation.
- **Spiritual connection:** Intuition connects you with your spirituality, guiding you on your path and bringing you closer to your divine essence.
- **Emotional well-being:** Intuition helps you make choices that promote your emotional well-being and happiness.
- **More authentic relationships:** Intuition helps you connect with people in a more authentic and profound way.

Exercise:

Take some time to connect with your intuition. Find a quiet place, close your eyes, and breathe deeply. Ask your inner self a question and patiently wait for the answer, without judgment or expectation. Write down your impressions, feelings, and insights in your journal.

Intuition is an inner compass that guides you towards your truth, your wisdom, and your life purpose. By learning to listen to this inner voice, you connect with your essence, make wiser decisions, and build a more authentic, meaningful, and fulfilling life.

Chapter 47
Synchronicity and the Law of Attraction

In the previous chapters, we learned to listen to the voice of intuition, the compass that guides us on our inner journey. Now, let's expand our perception and explore synchronicity and the Law of Attraction, concepts that reveal the profound interconnection between our thoughts, emotions, and the reality that surrounds us. We will discover how we can co-create our life, aligning our energy with the energy of the universe and manifesting our dreams and desires.

Imagine the universe as a great web of energy, where everything is interconnected and influences each other. Synchronicity is like a conductive thread in this web, connecting seemingly random events, people, and situations, revealing a deeper meaning and a greater purpose behind coincidences.

The Law of Attraction, in turn, teaches us that "like attracts like." Our thoughts, emotions, and beliefs act as magnets, attracting experiences and situations that vibrate at the same frequency into our reality. By cultivating positive thoughts, elevated emotions, and empowering beliefs, we pave the way for the manifestation of our dreams and desires.

Synchronicity and the Law of Attraction complement each other, revealing the co-creative nature of reality. By connecting with our intuition, cultivating positivity, and vibrating in tune with our desires, we enter a flow of synchronicities that lead us towards the realization of our dreams.

Co-creating reality:

- **Pay attention to synchronicities:** Be aware of events, people, and situations that seem like "meaningful coincidences." They may contain important messages from the universe, guiding you on your path and showing you that you are on the right track.
- **Cultivate positive thoughts:** Your thoughts are like seeds that you plant in the garden of your reality. Cultivate positive, constructive, and empowering thoughts, and you will reap the fruits of joy, abundance, and fulfillment.
- **Elevate your emotions:** Elevated emotions, such as love, gratitude, and joy, vibrate at a high frequency and attract positive experiences into your life. Practice gratitude daily, cultivate optimism, and connect with the joy of living.
- **Visualize your dreams:** Use creative visualization to imagine your dreams as if they were already real, feeling the emotions and sensations of having already achieved them. Visualization is a powerful tool for manifesting your desires.
- **Affirm your desires:** Declare your desires to the universe with clarity and conviction, using

positive affirmations that express your dreams and aspirations.
- **Act towards your goals:** The Law of Attraction doesn't just work with thoughts and emotions. It is necessary to act towards your goals, making decisions, making choices, and moving towards the realization of your dreams.
- **Trust the universe:** Have faith in the process, trust the wisdom of the universe, and believe that your dreams are manifesting in your life.
- **Be grateful:** Cultivate gratitude for everything you already have and for everything that is to come. Gratitude opens doors to abundance and attracts even more blessings into your life.

Benefits of understanding synchronicity and the Law of Attraction:
- **Co-creation of reality:** Empowers you to take control of your life and co-create your reality in a conscious and positive way.
- **Manifestation of dreams:** Helps you manifest your dreams and desires by aligning your energy with the energy of the universe.
- **Increased positivity:** Encourages you to cultivate positive thoughts, elevated emotions, and empowering beliefs.
- **Connection with the universe:** Connects you with the wisdom of the universe and shows you that you are part of something greater than yourself.
- **Life purpose:** Helps you find your life purpose and live with more meaning and fulfillment.

- **Integral well-being:** Promotes integral well-being, harmonizing body, mind, and spirit.
Exercise:

Pay attention to the synchronicities in your life. Write them down in a journal and reflect on their meaning. Cultivate positive thoughts, elevated emotions, and visualize your dreams as if they were already real. Affirm your desires to the universe with clarity and conviction.

You are a co-creator of your reality. By understanding synchronicity and the Law of Attraction, you become a conductor of your life, conducting the symphony of your dreams with mastery and manifesting the life you desire.

Chapter 48
Living in Harmony with the Universe

In the previous chapters, we explored synchronicity and the Law of Attraction, unraveling the co-creation of reality. Now, let's take a step further and discover how we can live in harmony with the universe, aligning our thoughts, emotions, and actions with the natural laws that govern life.

Imagine the universe as a great symphony, where each being, each element, each event vibrates at a unique frequency, contributing to the harmony of the whole. Living in harmony with the universe is like dancing to the rhythm of this cosmic symphony, tuning your energy with the energy of the whole and flowing in sync with the natural laws that govern life.

This harmony manifests itself on all levels of our being: in the physical body, through health and vitality; in the mind, through inner peace and mental clarity; in emotions, through balance and serenity; and in the spirit, through connection with the divine and life purpose.

Living in harmony with the universe is a process of self-knowledge, of alignment with your values and life purpose, and of respect for the natural laws that govern the universe. It is a path of growth, evolution, and expansion of consciousness, which leads you to a fuller, more authentic, and happier life.

Tuning in to the harmony of the universe:
- **Observe nature:** Nature is a mirror of the harmony of the universe. Observe the natural cycles, the rhythm of the seasons, the interdependence between living beings, and the beauty of creation. Be inspired by the wisdom of nature to live in harmony with the universe.
- **Cultivate respect:** Respect yourself, others, nature, and all forms of life. Recognize the interconnection between all beings and the importance of living in harmony with the planet.
- **Practice gratitude:** Cultivate gratitude for everything you have in your life, for the blessings you receive, and for the opportunities that present themselves. Gratitude connects you with the abundance of the universe and opens you to receive even more.
- **Follow your intuition:** Trust your intuition, that inner voice that guides you with wisdom and connects you with your deepest truth. Intuition is a channel of communication with the universe, which helps you make decisions aligned with your life purpose.
- **Live with purpose:** Find your life purpose and live according to it. Seek meaning in your actions, contribute to the good of the world, and leave your positive mark on the universe.

- **Be authentic:** Live according to your values and your inner truth. Be authentic in your relationships, in your choices, and in your actions.
- **Cultivate inner peace:** Practice meditation, mindfulness, and other relaxation techniques to calm the mind, reduce stress, and cultivate inner peace.
- **Forgive and let go:** Forgive yourself and others, releasing hurts, resentments, and guilt that may be blocking your energy flow and hindering your inner harmony.
- **Connect with your spirituality:** Cultivate your connection with the divine, whatever your belief or spiritual path. Spirituality connects you with something greater than yourself, giving you strength, hope, and purpose.
- **Accept challenges:** Life is a journey with challenges and obstacles. Accept challenges as opportunities for learning and growth, and trust that the universe supports and guides you on your path.

Benefits of living in harmony with the universe:

- **Inner peace and serenity:** Living in harmony with the universe gives you inner peace, serenity, and emotional balance.
- **Health and vitality:** Promotes physical health, vitality, and integral well-being.
- **Abundance and prosperity:** Opens doors to abundance, prosperity, and the fulfillment of your dreams.

- **Harmonious relationships:** Contributes to building more harmonious relationships based on love, respect, and understanding.
- **Life purpose:** Helps you find your life purpose and live with more meaning and fulfillment.
- **Spiritual connection:** Strengthens your connection with the divine and leads you to a deeper and more spiritualized life.

Exercise:

Reflect on how you can live in greater harmony with the universe. Observe nature, cultivate respect, gratitude, and inner peace. Follow your intuition, live with purpose, and connect with your spirituality.

Living in harmony with the universe is a path of self-knowledge, growth, and expansion of consciousness. By aligning yourself with the natural laws that govern life, you become a channel for the vital energy of the universe, manifesting health, abundance, inner peace, and happiness in your life.

Chapter 49
Prosperity and Abundance

In the previous chapters, we learned to live in harmony with the universe, attuning our energy to the natural flow of life. Now, let's explore prosperity and abundance, discovering how we can open our hearts and minds to receive the blessings that the universe has to offer us.

Imagine prosperity as an abundant river flowing towards you, bringing with it riches, opportunities, joy, and fulfillment. Abundance is a state of fullness, where you feel complete, grateful, and satisfied with everything life gives you.

Prosperity is not limited to material wealth, but encompasses all areas of life: health, love, relationships, happiness, inner peace, and life purpose. It is a state of grace where you feel connected to the inexhaustible source of blessings from the universe and open yourself to receive all the good that life has to offer.

Often, limiting beliefs, fears, and emotional blocks can prevent prosperity from flowing freely in your life. By identifying and transforming these obstacles, you pave the way for abundance in all areas of your life.

Opening yourself to prosperity and abundance:
- **Cultivate gratitude:** Gratitude is the key that opens the doors to abundance. Give thanks for everything you already have, for the small and big blessings that life offers you. By recognizing and appreciating the richness that already exists in your life, you attract even more prosperity.
- **Free yourself from limiting beliefs:** Identify and transform limiting beliefs about money, success, and worthiness. Replace thoughts of scarcity with beliefs of abundance, affirming that you are deserving of all the good things life has to offer.
- **Visualize prosperity:** Use creative visualization to imagine your life abundant in all areas: health, love, relationships, finances, career, and life purpose. Feel the emotions and sensations of already living this reality.
- **Act towards your goals:** Prosperity does not fall from the sky. Define your goals, create an action plan, and act towards achieving your dreams. The universe will support you in your efforts and guide you towards abundance.
- **Share your prosperity:** Share your blessings with others, whether through donations, volunteer work, or acts of generosity. By sharing your prosperity, you multiply it and contribute to creating a more abundant world for all.
- **Trust the universe:** Have faith in the process, trust in the abundance of the universe, and believe

that you are being guided and supported on your journey.
- **Cultivate self-esteem:** Recognize your worth, your talents, and your abilities. Believe in yourself and your potential to create a prosperous and abundant life.
- **Celebrate your achievements:** Acknowledge and celebrate each achievement, no matter how small. Celebration motivates you to keep growing and reach new levels of prosperity.
- **Stay focused:** Stay focused on your goals and your vision of prosperity, avoiding distractions and staying true to your purpose.
- **Be patient:** Prosperity manifests itself at the right time. Be patient, persistent, and trust that the universe is working in your favor.

Benefits of opening yourself to prosperity and abundance:
- **Fulfillment of dreams:** Attracts opportunities, resources, and synchronicities that propel you towards the fulfillment of your dreams.
- **Financial well-being:** Creates conditions for financial prosperity, attracting wealth, abundance, and material security.
- **Health and vitality:** Promotes physical health, vitality, and overall well-being.
- **Harmonious relationships:** Attracts healthy relationships based on love, respect, and reciprocity.
- **Inner peace and happiness:** Cultivates inner peace, gratitude, joy, and happiness.

- **Life purpose:** Helps you find your life purpose and live with more meaning and fulfillment.

Exercise:

Reflect on your beliefs about prosperity and abundance. Identify and transform limiting beliefs. Practice gratitude daily, visualize your abundant life, and act towards your goals.

Prosperity and abundance are divine rights of all beings. By opening your heart and mind to receive, you connect with the inexhaustible source of blessings from the universe and manifest the prosperous and abundant life you deserve.

Chapter 50
Awakening the Creative Potential

In the previous chapters, we sought harmony with the universe and opened the way to prosperity and abundance. Now, let's dive into the realm of creativity and inspiration, discovering how we can awaken the creative potential that resides in each of us and manifest beauty, innovation, and originality in our lives.

Imagine creativity as an inexhaustible source of ideas, an inner flame that illuminates the mind and drives innovation, art, and self-expression. Inspiration, in turn, is like the divine breath that feeds this flame, bringing insights, ideas, and the energy needed to bring your creations to life.

Creativity is not limited to the arts, but manifests itself in all areas of life: in problem-solving, communication, relationships, work, and the search for new solutions and perspectives. It is the ability to think outside the box, to connect ideas in an original way, and to give life to something new and unique.

Awakening the creative potential is like opening the doors of your imagination, freeing the creative energy that resides within you and allowing it to express itself fully. It is a process of self-knowledge, of connecting with your intuition and opening yourself to the inspiration that flows from the universe.

Awakening the creative potential:
- **Cultivate curiosity:** Be curious, explore the world around you, ask questions, seek new knowledge and experiences. Curiosity is the fuel of creativity, feeding the mind with new ideas and perspectives.
- **Free your imagination:** Give wings to your imagination, allowing it to fly freely without limits or judgments. Play with ideas, explore new possibilities, and allow yourself to daydream.
- **Connect with your intuition:** Intuition is the voice of your creativity, whispering ideas, insights, and innovative solutions. Quiet the mind, listen to your inner voice, and trust your creative instincts.
- **Seek inspiration:** Be inspired by other people, nature, art, music, literature, and everything that touches and moves you. Inspiration is like a breath of life that feeds the flame of creativity.
- **Experiment and explore:** Experiment with new techniques, materials, and forms of expression. Explore different areas of knowledge, step out of your comfort zone, and allow yourself to make mistakes and learn from them.
- **Create an inspiring environment:** Surround yourself with beauty, art, music, and colors that inspire and motivate you to create. Organize your workspace in a way that stimulates creativity and the flow of ideas.

- **Dedicate time to create:** Set aside time in your routine to dedicate to your creativity, whether it's painting, writing, dancing, playing a musical instrument, cooking, or any other activity that inspires you.
- **Share your creations:** Share your creations with the world, whether through exhibitions, presentations, publications, or simply sharing with friends and family. Sharing your creations connects you with others and inspires you to continue creating.
- **Believe in your potential:** Believe in your creative potential, recognize your talents and abilities, and trust in your ability to bring something new and unique to life.
- **Celebrate your creativity:** Celebrate every idea, every inspiration, every creation. Recognize the value of your creative expression and take pride in your accomplishments.

Benefits of awakening creativity and inspiration:
- **Self-knowledge:** Creativity connects you with your essence, revealing your talents, passions, and deepest potentials.
- **Innovation and problem-solving:** Increases your ability to find creative solutions to life's challenges.
- **Self-expression:** Allows you to express your individuality, your feelings, and your worldview in an authentic way.

- **Joy and fulfillment:** Creativity gives you joy, satisfaction, and a sense of personal fulfillment.
- **Connection with the universe:** Connects you with the creative energy of the universe, opening you to inspiration and intuition.
- **Emotional well-being:** Reduces stress, increases self-esteem, and promotes emotional well-being.

Exercise:

Take some time to awaken your creativity. Explore new activities, seek inspiration in nature and art, and allow yourself to express your individuality freely and authentically.

Creativity is a divine gift that resides in each of us. By awakening the creative potential, you connect with the inexhaustible source of inspiration from the universe and manifest beauty, innovation, and originality in your life.

Chapter 51
Expanding the Circle of Love

In the previous chapters, we explored the connection with the universe and the manifestation of prosperity. Now, let's expand our gaze beyond ourselves and discover the power of service to others and compassion, paths that connect us with humanity, nourish the soul, and open doors to a life richer in meaning and purpose.

Imagine love as a flame that expands with each gesture of compassion, each act of service, each hug of solidarity. Service to others is like the fuel that feeds this flame, radiating warmth, light, and hope to the world. Compassion, in turn, is the lens that allows us to see the other with empathy, understanding their pain, their joys, and their needs.

Serving others is dedicating your time, your talents, and your energies to contribute to the well-being of other people, the community, and the planet. It is an act of love in action, which transcends selfishness and connects us with the interdependence between all beings.

Compassion is the ability to put yourself in another's shoes, to feel their emotions, to understand their pain, and to offer support and solidarity. It is a balm that heals the wounds of the soul, promotes unity, and strengthens the bonds of love and fraternity.

Expanding the circle of love:
- **Cultivate empathy:** Practice active listening, seek to understand the perspectives and feelings of others, and put yourself in their shoes. Empathy is the basis of compassion and service to others.
- **Identify your skills and talents:** What are your gifts and talents? How can you use them to serve others and contribute to the good of the world?
- **Find causes that inspire you:** What social, environmental, or humanitarian causes touch you and motivate you to act? Find causes that resonate with your values and inspire you to dedicate your time and energy.
- **Offer help:** Offer help to those in need, whether through volunteer work, donations, acts of kindness, or simply offering a listening ear and a welcoming hug.
- **Practice kindness:** Be kind to the people around you, offering words of support, smiles, compliments, and gestures of affection. Kindness is an act of love that transforms the world.
- **Be an agent of change:** Be an agent of change in your community, participating in social projects, advocating for causes you believe in, or simply inspiring the people around you with your actions and attitudes.
- **Forgive and free yourself:** Forgiveness is an act of compassion that frees you and others from the

weight of anger, resentment, and guilt. Forgive yourself and others, and open space for love and healing.
- **Cultivate gratitude:** Give thanks for the opportunities to serve, for the people who cross your path, and for the blessings you receive. Gratitude connects you with the abundance of the universe and inspires you to share your love and compassion.
- **Connect with your spirituality:** Spirituality connects you with universal love, inspiring you to serve others and live with compassion and purpose.

Benefits of service to others and compassion:
- **Life purpose:** Finding meaning and purpose in your life, contributing to the good of the world and making a difference in people's lives.
- **Happiness and well-being:** Helping others increases feelings of happiness, well-being, and personal fulfillment.
- **Human connection:** Strengthens the bonds of human connection, promoting unity, solidarity, and love for others.
- **Personal growth:** Develops empathy, compassion, gratitude, and other virtues that make you a better person.
- **Physical and mental health:** Reduces stress, increases self-esteem, and promotes physical and mental health.
- **Expansion of consciousness:** Expands your consciousness, connecting you with the

interdependence between all beings and with universal love.

Exercise:

Identify a cause that inspires you and find ways to contribute to it. Offer help to those in need, practice kindness, and be an agent of change in your community.

Service to others and compassion are like bridges that connect us with humanity, nourish the soul, and open doors to a life richer in meaning, purpose, and love. By expanding the circle of love, you contribute to creating a more just, compassionate, and harmonious world.

Chapter 52
Awakening Cosmic Consciousness

In the previous chapters, we expanded the circle of love through service to others and compassion. Now, let's embark on a journey of expanding consciousness, awakening to cosmic consciousness and transcending the limits of individual perception.

Imagine cosmic consciousness as an infinite ocean of knowledge, wisdom, and interconnectedness, where each being, each planet, each star is a drop that makes up this vast ocean. Awakening cosmic consciousness is like diving into this ocean, expanding your horizons of perception and connecting with the unity that permeates all creation.

Cosmic consciousness transcends individuality, ego, and the limitations of the mind. It is the perception that we are part of something much greater than ourselves, interconnected with all beings and everything that exists in the universe. It is the understanding that life is a complex web of relationships, where every action, every thought, every emotion reverberates throughout the cosmos.

Awakening cosmic consciousness is like opening your eyes to a new reality, where separation dissolves and unity reveals itself in all its magnificence. It is a call to transcend the boundaries of the ego, connect with universal wisdom, and live in harmony with the cosmos.

Expanding the horizons of perception:

- **Connect with nature:** Nature is a portal to cosmic consciousness. Contemplate the vastness of the starry sky, the beauty of the mountains, the power of the sea, the delicacy of flowers. Feel the interconnection between all living beings and the vital energy that pulsates in every particle of the universe.
- **Practice meditation:** Meditation is a powerful tool to quiet the mind, expand consciousness, and connect with your divine essence. Through meditation, you can access deeper states of consciousness and open yourself to the perception of cosmic unity.
- **Study and learn:** Seek knowledge about cosmology, philosophy, spirituality, and other areas that help you understand the vastness of the universe and the interconnectedness of all things.
- **Cultivate compassion:** Compassion is the bridge that connects you with humanity and all living beings. By cultivating compassion, you recognize the unity that permeates all creation and open yourself to the experience of universal love.
- **Live with purpose:** Find your life purpose and live according to it. By contributing to the good of the world and serving others, you align yourself with the flow of life and become an agent of positive transformation in the universe.

- **Detach from the ego:** The ego is the illusion of separation, which limits you and prevents you from experiencing the fullness of cosmic consciousness. Practice detachment, humility, and surrender, and free yourself from the shackles of the ego to connect with the unity of the universe.
- **Trust your intuition:** Intuition is the voice of your soul, which guides you with wisdom and connects you with universal intelligence. Trust your instincts, follow your inner voice, and open yourself to the guidance of the universe.
- **Cultivate gratitude:** Give thanks for the gift of life, for the beauty of the universe, and for the opportunity to be part of this great cosmic journey. Gratitude connects you with the abundance of the universe and opens you to receive the blessings of life.
- **Be an observer:** Observe your thoughts, emotions, and actions with detachment and compassion. By becoming an observer of your own experience, you free yourself from the conditioning of the mind and open yourself to the perception of reality in its totality.

Benefits of awakening cosmic consciousness:
- **Expansion of perception:** Broadens your worldview, connecting you with the vastness of the universe and the interconnectedness of all things.
- **Inner peace and serenity:** Brings inner peace, serenity, and the understanding that you are part of something greater than yourself.

- **Life purpose:** Helps you find your life purpose and live with more meaning and fulfillment.
- **Compassion and universal love:** Awakens compassion, unconditional love, and connection with all beings.
- **Freedom and transcendence:** Frees you from the shackles of the ego and leads you to transcend your individuality.
- **Wisdom and intuition:** Connects you with universal wisdom and strengthens your intuition.
- **Integral well-being:** Promotes integral well-being, harmonizing body, mind, and spirit.

Exercise:

Connect with nature, practice meditation, cultivate compassion and detachment. Seek knowledge about the universe and trust your intuition. Live with purpose and gratitude, and open yourself to the experience of cosmic consciousness.

Awakening cosmic consciousness is a call to transcend the limits of your individual perception and connect with the unity that permeates all creation. It is a path of expansion, love, and wisdom that leads you to a fuller, more meaningful life connected to the universe.

Chapter 53
Living Fully

In the previous chapters, we expanded our awareness to the vast horizons of the cosmos. Now, let's turn our attention to the only moment that truly exists: the now. Let's explore the power of now, discovering how we can free ourselves from the shackles of the past and future, and live fully in the present moment.

Imagine time as a river flowing incessantly, carrying with it the past, present, and future. The past is gone, the future has not yet arrived, and the only real moment is now, this present instant that is renewed with each breath.

The mind, however, has a tendency to get lost in thoughts about the past, dwelling on memories, regrets, and hurts, or to project itself into the future, feeding anxieties, fears, and expectations. This mental wandering takes us away from the present moment, prevents us from experiencing life to the fullest, and imprisons us in cycles of suffering.

Living in the now is like anchoring your attention in the present moment, freeing yourself from the chains of the past and future, and opening yourself to the experience of life in its totality. It is being present in each breath, in each sensation, in each thought, in each emotion, without judgment or resistance.

The power of now lies in its ability to connect you with your essence, with your inner peace, and with the inexhaustible source of joy and vitality that resides within you. By living in the now, you free yourself from suffering, open yourself to the beauty of life, and experience the fullness of being.

Anchoring yourself in the present:
- **Pay attention to your breath:** Breathing is the anchor that connects you to the present moment. Notice the air entering and leaving your lungs, feel the movement of your body with each inhalation and exhalation.
- **Focus on your senses:** Pay attention to the sensations of your body, the sounds around you, the colors, smells, and tastes you experience. By connecting with your senses, you anchor yourself in the present moment and open yourself to the richness of sensory experience.
- **Observe your thoughts without identifying with them:** Your thoughts are like clouds passing through the sky of your mind. Observe them without judgment, without clinging to them or getting carried away by them. Simply observe them and let them go.
- **Practice gratitude:** Give thanks for the blessings of the present moment, for the little things that bring you joy, and for the lessons that life offers you. Gratitude connects you with the abundance of the now and opens you to the beauty of life.

- **Embrace emotions:** Allow yourself to feel your emotions without resistance or judgment. Embrace your joys, sorrows, anger, and fears, recognizing that they are part of the human experience and connect you with your authenticity.
- **Connect with your body:** Move, dance, practice yoga, walk in nature, do activities that bring you pleasure and connect you with the vitality of your body.
- **Simplify your life:** Let go of things, commitments, and relationships that no longer serve you. Simplify your life, creating space for what really matters and makes you happy.
- **Cultivate silence:** Set aside moments of silence and solitude to connect with your inner peace and listen to the voice of your intuition.
- **Be present in your relationships:** Dedicate quality time to the people you love, being present in body and soul in the moments you share.
- **Accept what is:** Accept the present moment as it is, without resistance or judgment. Trust the flow of life and open yourself to the infinite possibilities that the now offers you.

Benefits of living in the power of now:
- **Freedom and inner peace:** Free yourself from the shackles of the past and future, experiencing inner peace and the freedom to be who you truly are.

- **Increased joy and vitality:** Connect with the inexhaustible source of joy and vitality that resides within you.
- **Reduced stress and anxiety:** Decreases stress, anxiety, and suffering by freeing yourself from worries and fears.
- **Increased creativity and intuition:** Opens space for creativity, intuition, and inspiration to flow freely.
- **Improved relationships:** Strengthens bonds of connection with people, promoting authenticity and intimacy.
- **Fulfillment and accomplishment:** Experience life to the fullest, with gratitude, presence, and fulfillment.

Exercise:

Practice presence in your daily life. Focus on your breathing, your senses, your emotions, and your thoughts. Cultivate gratitude, embrace the present moment, and open yourself to the experience of life in its totality.

The power of now lies in its ability to connect you with your essence, with your inner peace, and with the inexhaustible source of joy and vitality that resides within you. By living in the now, you free yourself from suffering, open yourself to the beauty of life, and experience the fullness of being.

Chapter 54
A Conscious Lifestyle

In the previous chapters, we anchored our attention in the power of now, experiencing the fullness of the present moment. Now, let's integrate self-regression into our daily lives, transforming it into a conscious lifestyle, a path to continuous growth, inner harmony, and personal fulfillment.

Imagine self-regression as a guiding thread that accompanies you in every step of your journey, guiding you with wisdom, connecting you with your essence, and propelling you towards your best version. Integrating self-regression into everyday life is like weaving this thread into every moment of your life, transforming each experience into an opportunity for learning, growth, and self-knowledge.

Self-regression is not limited to specific moments of practice, such as meditation or relaxation. It manifests itself in every choice, in every thought, in every action, in every relationship. It is a state of presence, awareness, and connection with oneself, with others, and with the universe.

By integrating self-regression into your daily life, you transform your life into a journey of self-discovery, healing, and expansion of consciousness. You become the protagonist of your story, creating the reality you desire and living with more purpose, joy, and fulfillment.

Weaving self-regression into everyday life:
- **Start the day with intention:** When you wake up, take a few minutes to connect with your breath, give thanks for the blessings of life, and set your intentions for the day. What energy do you want to cultivate today? What are your goals and priorities?
- **Practice mindfulness:** Cultivate mindfulness in your daily activities, whether it's showering, walking, eating, working, or interacting with other people. Pay attention to your senses, your thoughts, and your emotions, anchoring yourself in the present moment.
- **Observe your thoughts and emotions:** Be aware of your thoughts and emotions throughout the day. Identify negative thought patterns, limiting beliefs, and challenging emotions, and use the tools of self-regression to transform them.
- **Communicate assertively:** Express your needs, desires, and limits clearly, respectfully, and authentically. Practice active listening and cultivate healthy relationships based on open communication and empathy.
- **Cultivate gratitude:** Find reasons to be grateful each day, no matter how small. Gratitude connects you to the abundance of the universe and opens you to receive the blessings of life.

- **Practice self-care:** Take time to take care of yourself, whether through healthy eating, exercise, restful sleep, contact with nature, or moments of relaxation and leisure.
- **Forgive and let go:** Practice forgiveness, releasing hurts, resentments, and guilt that may be weighing you down. Forgive yourself and others, and make room for healing and inner peace.
- **Connect with your spirituality:** Set aside time to nurture your spirituality, whether through meditation, prayer, reading sacred texts, or other practices that connect you with the divine.
- **Celebrate your achievements:** Acknowledge and celebrate your achievements, no matter how small. Celebration motivates you to keep growing and achieving your goals.
- **Learn from your mistakes:** See mistakes as opportunities for learning and growth. Don't blame or criticize yourself, but use challenging experiences as a springboard to evolve and strengthen yourself.

Benefits of integrating self-regression into everyday life:

- **Self-knowledge and personal growth:** Promotes self-knowledge, personal development, and the expansion of consciousness.
- **Balance and harmony:** Cultivates inner balance, harmony between body, mind, and spirit, and inner peace.
- **Resilience and inner strength:** Strengthens resilience, increases the ability to deal with

challenges, and makes you stronger in the face of adversity.
- **Healthy relationships:** Contributes to building healthier, more authentic, and meaningful relationships.
- **Personal and professional fulfillment:** Propels you towards the fulfillment of your dreams and goals, both in your personal and professional life.
- **Integral well-being:** Promotes integral well-being, physical and mental health, and authentic happiness.

Exercise:

Reflect on how you can integrate self-regression into your daily life. Choose a practice that resonates with you and start applying it in your everyday moments. Observe how this practice transforms your perception, your emotions, and your actions, and leads you to a more conscious and fulfilling life.

Self-regression is a path of self-discovery, healing, and transformation that accompanies you in every step of your journey. By integrating self-regression into your daily life, you weave the web of your life with threads of awareness, love, and wisdom, creating a more authentic, harmonious, and happy reality.

Chapter 55
Integrating Self-Regression into Life

We have reached the end of our self-regression journey, exploring a vast universe of techniques, concepts, and practices for self-knowledge, healing, and personal development. Now is the time to integrate these learnings into your life, transforming them into tools to build a more authentic, harmonious, and happy reality.

Throughout this course, we have traveled a path that has taken us from self-knowledge to connection with the universe, from managing emotions to awakening cosmic consciousness, from caring for the body to expanding the soul. We have learned to listen to the voice of intuition, to cultivate positivity, to overcome challenges with resilience, to manifest our dreams, and to live in harmony with the flow of life.

Self-regression is a never-ending journey, a constant search for self-knowledge, growth, and expansion of consciousness. It is an invitation to become the protagonist of your story, to take control of your life, and to create the reality you desire.

Integrating self-regression into life:
- **Practice consistently:** The key to success in self-regression is consistent practice. Incorporate the techniques and concepts you have learned into

your daily routine, devoting time to meditation, relaxation, visualization, self-knowledge, and connection with your spirituality.
- **Be patient and compassionate:** The journey of self-regression is a gradual process that requires time, patience, and self-compassion. Celebrate each step taken, forgive your mistakes, and embrace yourself with love and understanding.
- **Share your learnings:** Share your knowledge and experiences with other people, inspiring them to walk the path of self-regression and build a more conscious and happy life.
- **Continue learning:** Self-regression is an infinite universe of knowledge and wisdom. Continue seeking new learning, exploring different techniques, and deepening your connection with yourself, with others, and with the universe.
- **Trust your intuition:** Intuition is your inner compass, guiding you towards your truth and your life purpose. Trust your instincts, follow your inner voice, and open yourself to the wisdom that resides in your heart.
- **Live with purpose:** Find your life purpose and live according to it. Seek meaning in your actions, contribute to the good of the world, and leave your positive mark on the universe.
- **Cultivate gratitude:** Give thanks for the blessings of life, for the opportunities for learning and growth, and for all the people who accompany you on your journey. Gratitude

connects you to the abundance of the universe and opens you to receive even more.
- **Be authentic:** Live according to your values and your inner truth. Be authentic in your relationships, in your choices, and in your actions.
- **Cultivate inner peace:** Practice meditation, mindfulness, and other relaxation techniques to calm the mind, reduce stress, and cultivate inner peace.
- **Connect with the universe:** Cultivate your connection with the universe, whatever your belief or spiritual path. The connection with the universe gives you strength, hope, and the certainty that you are part of something greater than yourself.

Next steps:
- **Continue practicing self-regression techniques:** Maintain a daily routine of meditation, relaxation, visualization, and other practices that help you in self-knowledge, managing emotions, and connecting with your spirituality.
- **Seek to deepen your knowledge:** Explore books, courses, workshops, and other resources that help you deepen your knowledge of self-regression, personal development, and spirituality.
- **Share your learnings and inspire other people:** Share your self-regression journey with other people, inspiring them to seek self-knowledge, healing, and personal transformation.
- **Connect with a community:** Look for study groups, workshops, or online communities that

share your interests in self-regression and personal development. Sharing experiences and mutual support can strengthen your journey.
- **Seek professional help:** If you feel the need, seek the help of a qualified professional, such as a therapist, coach, or mentor, to assist you in your journey of self-knowledge and personal development.
- **Trust the process:** Trust the process of life, the synchronicities that guide you, and your ability to create the reality you desire. Have faith in yourself, in the universe, and in the power of love that drives you towards your best version.

Self-regression is a journey of transformation that invites you to awaken to your infinite potential, to live with more awareness, purpose, and fulfillment, and to co-create a more harmonious and happy reality for yourself and for the world. Continue on this path with courage, love, and wisdom, and celebrate the beauty of life in every step of your journey.

Epilogue

We have reached the end of this shared journey, and it is with deep gratitude that we say goodbye - but only temporarily, for we know that what you have experienced here will continue to echo in your life in many ways. The knowledge you have absorbed and the reflections that have awakened in your mind are now a part of you, ready to be applied, refined, and transformed into actions that resonate with your truth.

Thank you for trusting in every word, for allowing this book to find a place in your story. It is a privilege to be a part of your journey, even if only through these pages. We hope to have contributed in some way to illuminating your doubts, strengthening your courage, and inspiring a continuous search for balance and authenticity.

But more important than any teaching shared here is your ability to continue. The journey does not end with a book, a learning experience, or a moment of discovery. It continues because you continue, expanding and exploring new ways of being, feeling, and living.

Therefore, we encourage you to cultivate the curiosity that brought you here. Continue questioning, learning, and connecting with what makes sense for your growth. Allow yourself to revisit these pages, if necessary, or move on in search of other paths, other voices, other perspectives that resonate with what you have become throughout this process.

Remember that progress is not about always getting it right, but about staying committed to your evolution. Celebrate each small step forward and be kind to yourself in the inevitable pauses and restarts. Learning is continuous, and each step, however small it may seem, is an achievement towards your purpose.

Thank you for sharing this moment, for allowing us to be a part of your story. May the insights and tools presented here be seeds that blossom at the right time, bringing strength, clarity, and harmony along the way.

May this farewell be, in fact, an incentive for you to continue exploring your essence, venturing into the unknown, and discovering the extraordinary that lies within yourself.

And, with gratitude and hope, we leave one last wish: that you take with you not only the lessons, but also the certainty that the power to transform your life is, and always has been, in your hands.

www.ingramcontent.com/pod-product-compliance
Lightning Source LLC
LaVergne TN
LVHW041938070526
838199LV00051BA/2830